The New Pediatric Guide to Drugs and Vitamins

The New Pediatric Guide to Drugs and Vitamins

by Edward R. Brace and
Kenneth Anderson

Preface by
John P. Pacanowski, M.D.

A Stonesong Press Book

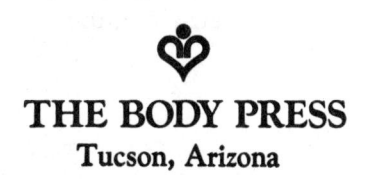

THE BODY PRESS
Tucson, Arizona

Copyright © 1982, 1987 by The Stonesong Press, Inc.

THE BODY PRESS
A division of HPBooks, Inc.
575 East River Road
Tucson, Arizona 85704

All rights reserved. No part of this book may be reproduced or transmitted in any form or by any means, electronic or mechanical, including photocopying, recording or by any information storage and retrieval system, without the written permission of the Publisher, except where permitted by law.

Manufactured in the United States of America

Library of Congress Cataloging in Publication Data

Brace, Edward R.
  The new pediatric guide to drugs & vitamins.

  Rev. ed. of: The pediatric guide to drugs and vitamins. 1982.
  Includes index.

  1. Drugs. 2. Vitamins. 3. Pediatric pharmacology.
I. Anderson, Kenneth, 1921-   . II. Brace,
Edward R. The pediatric guide to drugs and vitamins.
III. Title. [DNLM: 1. Drug Therapy—in infancy &
childhood—handbooks. 2. Vitamins—handbooks.
WS 39 B796n]

RJ560.B7   1987   615'.1 '088054   86 71875
ISBN 0-89586-538-6
ISBN 0-89586-528-9 (pbk.)

10 9 8 7 6 5 4 3 2
First Printing

Contents

To The Reader 7

Preface 8

Introduction 13

Alphabetical Description of Prescription
    and Over-the-Counter Drugs 19

Vitamins 265

List of Drugs by Primary Therapeutic
    Category 279

Index 283

To The Reader

WARNING

The information on drug products that is contained in this book—particularly in the section in each entry that mentions Children's Dosage—is not meant to be used by parents or other concerned adults to treat children. *Only a physician is qualified to diagnose and treat a child with a specific medical problem.* He or she will prescribe the appropriate medication in a form and dosage that is best for each individual child.

Keep all medications out of the reach of children! Overdosage can be fatal. Too many tragic examples exist of children being poisoned by drugs that have been left within easy reach—for example, aspirin poisoning is far too frequent in children. Never trust "child-proof" tops on drug bottles.

Household measures, such as teaspoons or tablespoons, are not precise. For example, teaspoons are manufactured in various sizes and may hold from three to five milliliters (ml) of liquid. When giving children liquid measures of a medication, do not take unnecessary chances in giving too little or too much. Ask your pharmacist for a professional measuring spoon.

Preface

Little in the human experience can extract more emotion than a sick or injured child. The young seem to become ill more frequently and to do so more rapidly than adults. They also suffer more accidental injuries—which, for the most part, fortunately are minor. Balancing this is the speed with which a child recovers. Children's bones knit more rapidly, their fevers come down more abruptly, and their convalescence is usually shorter. With proper treatment, including medication when necessary, illnesses pass as quickly as they come.

Perhaps the most important factor in the care of an ill child is the emotional input of the parents: the overwhelming need to have the child active and happy. Getting a youngster well, however, requires the efforts of several people: the researcher who looks for the better way to do it, the physician who diagnoses and prescribes, the industry that provides effective medications, and the many other health professionals are all part of the team.

Recently a new component has entered the spectrum of health care. As our society becomes more knowledgeable about health-care practices, we need ready sources of information about medications, laboratory tests, and treatments. Today's parents want to know what they are giving their child when they are using a prescription or an over-the-counter (OTC) drug. They quite properly consider this information to be their right.

Parents should assume the responsibility of knowing what medication is used and why. Being alert to possible side effects helps protect the child from potentially serious drug-induced reactions. Infants and small children cannot make decisions about what's being given to them (although they may try, especially if they don't like the taste). The burden rests on the informed adults around them.

The Pediatric Guide to Drugs and Vitamins is meant to help fulfill a portion of the responsibility that parents assume as they care for an ill child. The intent is to make parents aware of the major characteristics and possible complications of therapeutic agents.

This book does not attempt to be inclusive in the description of drugs. Only the most important points have been discussed. These are meant to alert parents to the possibility that the continued use of a medication or use of the wrong medication may cause the child difficulties. Above all, *this book is not a home-treatment manual.* The decision as to which and how much of a drug to use remains with the physician. He or she will use an approach based on years of experience as well as a wide variety of other factors.

The type of antibiotic a doctor prescribes for an infeciton, for example, depends on the age and size of the child as well as on the diagnosis of the illness. Children are not simply prewashed and preshrunk adults. Their metabolisms are different, and they require special dosage alterations. The significance of symptoms may also be considerably different in a child than in an adult whose body defenses are mature.

Years of experience and research have come up with a "drug of choice" for most diseases. When exact information is needed to treat an infection, "cultures" can be made to identify the offending bacteria. Further tests will show which of several antibiotics is most effective in killing the specific type of bacteria or arresting the course of the disease.

For problems that are not infections, doctors select medications based on what has been tested extensively and thought to be the most effective means of treatment. This information appears in the medical literature your physician has at his or her disposal. New agents are added when their safety and efficacy have been determined. Similarly, when experience indicates that an agent is either not beneficial or presents side effects that had not previously been recognized, it is removed from the drug market.

We are fortunate to have available to us a wide range of medications. At times, however, we all probably have some reluctance about using a "drug" for an illness, perhaps just because of the meaning that the word now conveys. We don't like to be ill, and we don't want our children ill. Further, we don't want to add additional risks from medicines to what is already going on with an illness. As understandable as these feelings might be, a medication that is known to be effective—when it is given for the proper reason and in the proper manner (amount, frequency, duration)—can be lifesaving.

When your child is ill and has been examined by a physician, it is proper to ask the doctor what the diagnosis is. It is also important to ask about the medication that will be prescribed. Parents should know the name of the drug, how to give it to the child, and when to expect some positive results from the treat- ment. Parents should also ask the physician what they should do if something unexpected arises. Most physicians are happy to provide this type of information, since it may help prevent a serious drug reaction or the development of a more serious illness than the one that was originally diagnosed.

Armed with the knowledge of what you are going to do, try to gain additional facts about the drugs your child takes. From either your pharmacist or the entries in this book, learn what the possible side effects are. Also, become familiar with what might be potentially serious adverse reactions. If your child develops suspicious signs and symptoms that might be related to the use of a prescription drug, ask the child's physician about the advisability of discontinuing use of the medication as soon as possible.

If your child ever does have a reaction to a drug, record the event in your medical records at home. Note the child's age, the name of the medication, and exactly what the reaction was. Imagine how frustrating it would be for a physician to have to prescribe a drug for an illness after hearing, "Yes, Jimmy had some sort of a problem, maybe a rash, after taking a thick pink liquid a long time ago." The exact details of any reaction should be recorded, safely kept, and available whenever your child is seen for an illness.

To achieve the desired benefits from therapy, it must be emphasized that any medication must be properly administered by the parents and a close watch kept on the child while he or she takes it. Prescription drugs should be taken at the times and in the exact amounts that are directed by the physician. More often than one would expect, various mistakes are made in following dosage instructions that cancel out or reduce the effectiveness of a drug.

Perhaps the most common error made by parents is discontinuing the use of a medication before the full prescription is given to a child. When the fever is gone and the child's behavior has returned to normal, it's easy to forget dosages or even to make the conscious decision to stop giving the medicaaf05—ion entirely. *This should never be done!* Antibiotic treatment for strep throat, for example, is not simply meant to clear up the symptoms of a sore throat. It is intended to prevent the development of rheumatic fever, and a *full ten-day course of therapy is needed.*

Antibiotics prescribed for an ear infection have a wider purpose than the relief of pain or the resolution of a fever. The drug is meant to prevent complications such as meningitis (inflammation of the membranes that cover the brain). It is important, then, to have the child complete the full course of therapy.

Extending the use of a medication for a longer period than was directed can also be harmful. Long-term use (in excess of the usual period of treatment) increases the likelihood of adverse reactions to the drug.

Dosage schedules are important as well. How effectively a medication works is based on maintaining an appropriate level of the drug in the circulating blood. That level can be achieved only if the drug is administered exactly as directed by the physician. For example, "every six hours" is not the same as "four times a day." In the latter case, the drug may be given in the morning, at noon, in the afternoon, and at bedtime (approximately every four hours), whereas in the former case, the drug must literally be given at intervals of every six hours. If a dose is forgotten, "doubling up" the next time might be dangerous. Follow the physician's directions carefully!

Unless you are advised otherwise by the child's doctor, always discard any unused medication. Saving it for the next illness or giving it to a neighbor to treat her child may cause serious problems.

Drugs have expiration dates and should be used within a given interval of time. Never use an old prescription drug to treat an illness for which the drug was not intended. A drug that was prescribed in the past for cramping stomach pain and diarrhea should not be used the next time without medical advice. One could inadvertently alter the symptoms and delay the diagnosis of a more serious illness, such as appendicitis. Similarly, giving one child's drug to another for what seems like the same type of illness may result in partial or inadequate treatment of a potentially dangerous condition.

Unlike friends or warm sunshine, more of a drug is not necessarily better. Giving a child twice as much of a medication won't get him or her better twice as fast. At the very least it's wasteful and expensive; but it may also be harmful if toxic (poisonous) levels are reached. Again, the frequent caution: Give the child the prescribed amount at the prescribed dosage schedule.

Included in *The Pediatric Guide to Drugs and Vitamins* are the most common non-prescription, or over-the-counter, drugs.

These are medications that are thought to have a wide enough margin of safety that they can be used without a physician's supervision. With these, as with prescription drugs, very careful guidelines must be followed. Use them only as directed on the package or label. If no improvement is noted in the child's condition, or if symptoms worsen, a physician must be consulted.

Finally, a few words about how medications fit into the overall physical and emotional health of a child. Some who have analyzed the frightening abuse of mind-altering drugs in our society have questioned the easy advertisement and availability of medications as a forerunner of misuse.

As soon as children can understand, they should be told exactly *what* they are being given as well as *why* it's being given. Don't simply say, "Take this, it will make you feel better." Say, "It's penicillin to kill the strep germ." Or, "It's aspirin to bring down your fever." We don't want the young to believe that when they feel bad all they have to do is take a pill to make the problem go away. Explain to children that pharmaceutical products (both prescription and non-prescription drugs) provide an artificial means of temporarily assisting the body in getting over a specific difficulty.

> John P. Pacanowski, M.D., F.A.A.P
> **Chief, Section of Pediatrics**
> **Guthrie Clinic Ltd.**
> **Sayre, Pennsylvania**

Introduction

Until the first edition of *The Pediatric Guide to Drugs and Vitamins* in 1982, no general reference book had been available to parents and other concerned adults that presented clear and concise information on the major groups of pharmaceutical products and dietary supplements that physicians prescribe for infants and children. It provided essential information about a wide variety of prescription drugs as well as about products that are freely available without a doctor's prescription (over-the-counter, or OTC, drugs). Because of the increasing number of drugs on the market, and because of the ever-changing formulations of those already available, this new edition has grown in coverage since the first edition as newly introduced drugs have gained in popularity of use. The need for a new edition nonetheless should make it clear that although every effort has been made to ensure accuracy and completeness, new information is as current and accurate as the latest information allows. Thus no claim is made that all possible side effects, adverse reactions or interactions with other drugs or substances are included.

To permit parents to check quickly on a specific drug product, all entries are listed in strict alphabetical order. Under the name of each drug will be found information on its generic (or chemical) name, its therapeutic category, available dosage forms, why the drug is used, the usual dosage for children, specific precautions and warnings associated with the use of the drug, and possible side effects that may be experienced by some children taking the product.

Most drugs are listed under their brand names. In a few instances, however, the generic name is listed in alphabetical order, with representative major brands mentioned under the listing.

Parents are cautioned not to continue using over-the-counter (non-prescription) drugs to treat a child for other than minor ailments. If the child fails to improve within a short time or if the symptoms become worse, consult a physician. Used properly, non-prescription drugs play an important role in preventing or minimizing the symptoms of relatively minor illnesses. Misused, they can mask the progress of a potentially serious underlying medical problem.

Never give a child more of a non-prescription drug than the label recommends. In some cases, a physician may suggest that a child use a non-prescription drug (indicated in this book by the letters OTC after the name of the product). In such instances, follow the dosage instructions of the physician.

Drugs that are available only with the prescription of a physician are usually much more potent than over-the-counter products. Because of this, it is essential to give the child the drug exactly as instructed. Exceeding the prescribed dosage could lead to potentially serious side effects. In some cases, a child may experience side effects at the recommended dosage. Should this occur, check with the physician immediately. It may be necessary to adjust the dosage or substitute another drug that is better tolerated by the child. Only the physician can make this decision.

Possible side effects have been listed for each prescription and non-prescription (OTC) drug that is discussed here. It is important for parents to realize that not every child taking a particular drug will experience one or more of these side effects. In most cases there will be no problem at all.

If the product is available without a prescription, it is wise to discontinue its use if a child experiences adverse effects. If it is a prescription drug, be sure to call the prescribing physician and report any evidence of the listed drug-induced side effects. In rare cases, a drug may cause side effects that are a direct threat to life. If the child is under close medical supervision during the course of an illness, these early signs and symptoms of drug toxicity can be recognized and measures taken by the physician to modify therapy.

The Pediatric Guide to Drugs and Vitamins provides up-to-date information on the use of drug products for infants, children, and adolescents. It does not contain information directed toward the adult patient or mention the dosage forms that are usually prescribed *only* for adults.

DOSAGE

When physicians prescribe drugs for infants and children, they are well aware that they are not merely dealing with "miniature adults." That is, effective therapy is not always a case of prescribing *less* of a certain drug but of understanding the possible therapeutic benefits and the potentially adverse effects on the not yet fully developed physiological system. The potential hazards are even greater when prescribing drugs for the newborn or premature infant.

Many physicians use a "conversion factor" to obtain pediatric dosages, based on the child's body weight in relation to the amount of drug given, usually in milligrams per kilogram of body weight. (1 kilogram = 2.2 pounds, and 1 milligram = 1/30,000th of an ounce.) In measuring dosage of some drugs, the term *lean* body weight, or *ideal* body weight, may be specified because including the extra weight contributed by body fat could result in dose sizes that are excessive for the child. For other drugs, the dosage may be based on the surface area of the child's body, so that a tall slim child and a short obese child may require the same drug dosage, regardless of their ages and body weights.

Parents have the right to know more about the drugs that are prescribed for their children—what they are designed to do and what possible side effects may occur in a few children taking them. Knowledgeable parents can be of great help to the child's doctor. Together, they form a team with a common goal—the prompt recovery of the ill child to normal health.

ASPIRIN AND REYE'S SYNDROME

In 1982, the U.S. Department of Health and Human Services issued a warning that giving aspirin to children under the age of sixteen with influenza ("flu") or chicken pox (varicella) increased the risk of developing Reye's syndrome, a rare but dangerous disease marked by encephalopathy (a "swelled" brain disorder) and fatty degeneration of the liver and kidneys. In recent years, the warning has been extended by some concerned physicians to include all children through the age of eighteen who may show symptoms of, or be recovering from, any virus infection, including infectious mononucleosis ("kissing disease") and the enteroviruses that may invade the digestive tract, causing gastroenteritis and other disorders.

The risk is small, the cause of Reye's syndrome is unknown, and the relationship between aspirin (and other salicylates) and Reye's syndrome is unclear. Considering that there are other nonprescription medical products available for the relief of pain and fever in children, if there is any uncertainty as to whether or not your child is suffering from viral illness, avoid it. Accordingly, we have included an "aspirin alert" in all those entries where aspirin and other salicylates are present.

Reye's syndrome symptoms usually include headache, vomiting, and mental or behavioral changes, such as stupor or coma.

Death may occur. Medical tests may find signs of swelling and fluid accumulation in the brain and fatty accumulations in the liver, heart, pancreas, spleen, kidneys, and lymph nodes. There is no specific treatment for Reye's syndrome and the outlook for recovery depends upon the severity of the symptoms.

Defenders of aspirin cite a lack of evidence of a direct, or cause-and-effect, relationship between aspirin and Reye's syndrome and that withholding aspirin will protect a child from the disease. Also, for many other childhood disorders, aspirin is still the cheapest, safest, and most widely-used over-the-counter (OTC) product for treating pain and inflammation. Acetaminophen, the main OTC alternative to aspirin, works in a way similar to aspirin. Ibuprofen is a second alternative but its use is not recommended for children under the age of twelve. Both interfere with the body's production of prostaglandin, a substance naturally present in tissue cells that causes an increase in pain and discomfort from an infection. Aspirin stops prostaglandin production while acetaminophen usually reduces production to a more tolerable level. For most mild cases of pain, the two OTC analgesics are equivalent. For severe pain, fever, or inflammation, more potent drugs are usually required with a doctor's prescription.

Acetaminophen does not have the anti-inflammatory effects of aspirin. But both work approximately the same way in reducing fever—by acting on the brain's temperature-regulating "thermostat." However, large doses of aspirin can have an adverse effect on the body's thermostat and cause even higher fever. Other potential hazards are its effects on blood clotting and damage to the lining of the stomach. Aspirin is technically an acid (acetylsalicylic acid), and when it is added to the natural acidity of the stomach, the lining of the stomach may be damaged. And because it interferes with blood clotting, aspirin, unless taken with an adequate amount of milk, water, or food, can produce small bleeding wounds in the stomach. "Buffered" forms of aspirin contain a substance to reduce the level of acidity in the stomach. Other, specially coated aspirin products are designed to be acid-resistant so they can pass through the stomach without dissolving, finally releasing the aspirin dose in the small intestine, where it can be absorbed directly into the bloodstream.

The major adverse effect of acetaminophen products is liver damage, because the liver converts acetaminophen into another chemical that destroys the liver cell membranes. However, this is unlikely unless excessive amounts of acetaminophen are used. While ibuprofen is anti-inflammatory, reduces fever, and relieves pain, like aspirin, it is not recommended as a substitute drug for people who are allergic to aspirin. Although the drug does not contain salicylates, it can provoke the same adverse reactions in those who are sensitive to aspirin.

The "jury is still out" on a relationship between aspirin use in children and Reye's Syndrome; the reader is advised to consult with the child's physician before giving any aspirin product.

VITAMINS

Information on vitamins is presented in a special section at the back of this book. If parents provide their children nutritionally balanced meals, selected from a variety of interesting foods or flavors, there is little need for vitamin supplements. However, many experts in nutrition feel that children, as well as adults, are often "cheated" in their intake of natural vitamins because they do not eat ideally balanced meals containing all the essential nutrients. Also, heavily processed foods and home preparation (prolonged freezing and overcooking) frequently rob food of its natural vitamins.

Most physicians recommend dietary supplements (in liquid form) of vitamins A, C, and D for babies. Mother's milk is generally deficient in vitamin D, although it may contain adequate amounts of vitamin C—particularly if the nursing mother eats plenty of fresh fruits and green leafy vegetables and drinks generous quantities of citrus juices.

A leading practicing pediatrician at the Guthrie Clinic, who is a fellow of the American Academy of Pediatrics and a clinical assistant professor of pediatrics at the State University of New York at Binghamton, assisted in the selection of the nearly 240 drugs that are most frequently prescribed or recommended in treating diseases and disorders of infancy and childhood. Each entry represents the most up-to-date medical information and general prescribing habits of physicians throughout the United States. However, new products are announced almost daily. Thus, a drug listed in this book may not be available because it has been discontinued, reformulated, or repackaged under a different brand name. Or a product may not be included because it has just been approved, discontinued (but supplies are still available), or other reasons. Also, product availability may vary from one region to another because of state laws, such as in drugs containing phenobarbital. Such drugs require a doctor's prescription in some states but not in others, and variations of the same product may exist in order to conform with different state laws.

Many of the entries in this book are *representative* products available without a doctor's prescription. These over-the-counter (OTC) drugs are typical of dozens of similar products that contain the same active ingredients. The inclusion of a particular OTC drug is not meant to imply it is the best one available. (Any drug listed in this book should not be considered an endorsement of the product by the authors, their consultants, or the publisher.) The general index at the back of this book lists the drugs by both brand name and generic name. By checking this index the reader can identify the major active ingredients in a particular drug and then compare them with similar products that may not be included in this book.

The ingredients listed under the generic names of the drugs represent only the *active* ingredients. Consumers should be aware that most pharmaceutical products also contain substances called *excipients*: these are generally harmless and therefore are not identified. They include artificial flavorings and colorings, sugar, starch, casein, oils, fats, waxes, or other materials that may help a tablet hold its shape, to make it dissolve faster after it is swallowed, or (with timed-release drugs) to protect it from being dissolved too quickly. A child may be allergic to the excipient rather than the active ingredient of the drug. Parents should be aware of the inactive ingredients in a drug, as well as the active ingredients, and should advise the doctor if the child has an allergy to an excipient.

The Pediatric Guide to Drugs and Vitamins should be used by parents only as a source of general information concerning drugs and the usual dosage for children. Only a physician can determine the best therapeutic approach in treating an individual child and determine the most effective dosage.

Alphabetical Description of Prescription and Over-The-Counter Drugs

Actifed® (OTC)

GENERIC NAME
This product contains a combination of triprolidine hydrochloride and pseudoephedrine hydrochloride.

PRODUCT CATEGORY
Antihistamine/decongestant.

DOSAGE FORM
Syrup and tablets.

WHY USED
It is used mainly to relieve the symptoms of hay fever (allergic rhinitis), including stuffy nose (nasal congestion), mild itching, and swelling.

CHILDREN'S DOSAGE
The usual dose for children age twelve and older is one tablet two or three times a day; children age six to twelve are given one half tablet three times a day. Children below the age of six are usually given the syrup form of Actifed. The following table lists the usual dosage of Actifed Syrup:

Age of Child	Teaspoonfuls (5 ml) 3 Times Daily
6 years and over	2
4 months–6 years	1
Under 4 months	½

The manufacturer recommends that the prescribing physician adjust the dosage according to the needs and the response of the child.

PRECAUTIONS AND WARNINGS
Actifed should not be given to newborn or premature infants or used to treat children who have asthma or other disorders of the lower part of the respiratory tract. Do not give Actifed to children who are hypersensitive (allergic) to antihistamines.

Actifed should be given with extreme caution (if at all) to children with diabetes.

POSSIBLE SIDE EFFECTS
The most commonly reported side effects include sedation, drowsiness, disturbed coordination, dizziness, and a thickening of secretions in the lower air passages (bronchial tubes). The nose, mouth, and throat may become excessively dry.

Actifed contains an antihistamine (triprolidine). In infants and children an overdosage of antihistamine may cause hallucinations, convulsions, or even death.

Actifed-C® Expectorant

GENERIC NAME
This product contains in each teaspoonful (5 ml) a combination of codeine phosphate (10 mg), guaifenesin (100 mg), pseudoephedrine hydrochloride (30 mg), and triprolidine hydrochloride (2 mg).

PRODUCT CATEGORY
Antitussive (cough suppressant)/expectorant/decongestant/antihistamine.

DOSAGE FORM
Syrup.

WHY PRESCRIBED
It is used to provide symptomatic relief of coughing in conditions such as the common cold, acute bronchitis, allergic asthma, croup, and emphysema.

CHILDREN'S DOSAGE

Age of Child	Teaspoonfuls (5 ml) 3-4 Times Daily
12 years and over	2
6–12 years	1
2–6 years	½

PRECAUTIONS AND WARNINGS
Codeine, the narcotic component of ingredient Actifed-C Expectorant may be habit-forming, especially if it is taken in excessive amounts for prolonged periods.

This product contains an antihistamine (triprolidine hydrochloride). An overdosage of antihistamine in infants and children can cause hallucinations, convulsions, or even death.

Actifed-C Expectorant should be used with caution in children with bronchial asthma, heart disease, thyroid disease, or high blood pressure (hypertension).

POSSIBLE SIDE EFFECTS
The most commonly reported side effects include mild stimulation, sedation, dizziness, disturbed coordination, thickening of secretions in the lower air passages (bronchial tubes), and excessive dryness of the nose, mouth, and throat. More rarely, a child may experience fluttering or rapid beating of the heart, extreme nervousness, blurred vision, hallucinations, or convulsions.

Agoral® (OTC)

GENERIC NAME
Agoral Plain contains mineral oil in a homogenized emulsion with agar, tragacanth, acacia, egg albumin, glycerin, and water. In addition, Agoral Raspberry and Agoral Marshmallow contain phenolphthalein.

PRODUCT CATEGORY
Laxative.

DOSAGE FORM
Liquid emulsion.

WHY USED
It is used to relieve constipation.

CHILDREN'S DOSAGE
Agoral is available without a doctor's prescription. Administer to children exactly as the label recommends. The usual recommended dosage for children over the age of six, in teaspoonfuls (5 ml) at bedtime:

Agoral Plain (without phenolphthalein)	2 to 4
Agoral Raspberry	1 to 2
Agoral Marshmallow	1 to 2

The medication can be taken alone or with water, milk, or fruit juice.

PRECAUTIONS AND WARNINGS
The mineral oil in Agoral lubricates the intestines in children who are constipated, thus helping reduce straining during bowel movements. Agoral Raspberry and Agoral Marshmallow also contain a laxative (phenolphthalein) that stimulates the wavelike (peristaltic) movements of the intestines. Such harsh-action laxatives are not recommended by many pediatricians for use in young children. In addition, some children may be allergic to phenolphthalein.

Do not give a child any laxative in the presence of abdominal pain, high fever, or nausea and vomiting. In such cases consult a physician.

The overuse of laxatives can aggravate constipation or even create the condition where it did not previously exist. Do not give a child laxatives regularly for more than one or two weeks without seeking medical advice. Although it is rare, the problem may be related to partial obstruction of the intestines and demands prompt medical diagnosis and treatment.

Constipation in infants is often associated with dietary habits, such as ingesting large amounts of milk.

POSSIBLE SIDE EFFECTS
Agoral Plain, used as directed, is relatively free from significant side effects. The phenolphthalein ingredient in Agoral Raspberry and Agoral Marshmallow may cause painful abdominal cramps in some children. A few children may also be allergic to this ingredient.

Allerest® (OTC)

GENERIC NAME
This product contains a combination of chlorpheniramine maleate and phenylpropanolamine. (Allerest Headache Strength and Allerest Sinus Pain Formula also contain acetaminophen.)

PRODUCT CATEGORY
Antihistamine/decongestant.

DOSAGE FORM
Chewable tablets (tablets and capsule forms are also available).

WHY USED
It is used to relieve the symptoms of hay fever (allergic rhinitis), including stuffy nose (nasal congestion), mild itching, running nose, and itching and watering eyes.

CHILDREN'S DOSAGE
Allerest is available without a doctor's prescription. Administer to children exactly as recommended on the label; the instructions may vary somewhat with the specific Allerest product.

PRECAUTIONS AND WARNINGS
Unless recommended by a physician, Allerest should not be used by children with heart disorders or diabetes. Do not give this drug to a child who is hypersensitive (allergic) to either of the ingredients.

If the child is under medical care, do not give him or her any drug without the knowledge and approval of the doctor.

POSSIBLE SIDE EFFECTS
Children taking Allerest may experience drowsiness, dizziness, nervousness, and excitability.

Ambenyl® Cough Syrup

GENERIC NAME
This product contains in each teaspoonful (5 ml) a combination of codeine phosphate (10 mg), bromodiphenhydramine hydrochloride (12.5 mg), and alcohol (5 percent).

PRODUCT CATEGORY
Antitussive (cough suppressant)/antihistamine.

DOSAGE FORM
Syrup.

WHY PRESCRIBED
It is used for the relief of upper air passage symptoms and coughs associated with the common cold or allergies.

CHILDREN'S DOSAGE
The usual dosage for children between the ages of six and twelve years is one-half to one teaspoonful every six hours. The product is not recommended for children under the age of six years.

PRECAUTIONS AND WARNINGS
Codeine, the narcotic components of this product may be habit-forming, especially if it is taken in excessive amounts for prolonged periods. Codeine overdosage can be fatal in young children.

Ambenyl Cough Syrup contains an antihistamine. An overdosage of antihistamine in infants and children can cause hallucinations, convulsions, or even death.

This product should be used with caution (if at all) in children with asthma, heart disease, hyperthyroid disease, or hypertension.

POSSIBLE SIDE EFFECTS
This "fixed-combination" drug can cause a wide variety of side effects. Among these are drowsiness; nervousness; confusion; nausea; vomiting; blurred vision; diarrhea; constipation; headache; drug-induced rashes or hives (urticaria); thickening of secretions in the lower air passages (bronchial tubes); dryness of the nose, mouth, and throat; and difficulty urinating.

Much less commonly, the side effects may include a drop in blood pressure (hypotension) and a severe form of anemia (hemolytic anemia).

Ambenyl®-D

GENERIC NAME
This product contains the following active ingredients: per each two teaspoonfuls (10 ml) guaifenesin (200 mg), pseudoephedrine hydrochloride (60 mg), and dextromethorphan hydrobromide (30 mg).

PRODUCT CATEGORY
Antitussive (cough suppressant)/expectorant/nasal decongestant.

DOSAGE FORM
Syrup.

WHY PRESCRIBED
It is used for the temporary relief of symptoms of nasal congestion due to the common cold or sinusitis and to help loosen secretions and suppress coughing associated with the common cold.

CHILDREN'S DOSAGE
The usual dosage for children between the ages of six and twelve years is two teaspoonfuls (10 ml) every six hours, and for children between two and six years one teaspoonful (5 ml) every six hours. The product should not be given to children under the age of two years unless authorized by a physician. No more than four doses should be given a child in any 24-hour period.

PRECAUTIONS AND WARNINGS
This product should not be used to relieve coughing symptoms associated with a chronic respiratory disorder such as asthma or emphysema, or in cases of excessive production of secretions in the air passages, except as authorized by a physician. A persistent cough may be a sign of a serious condition requiring a doctor's care.

Do not give the product to a child with diabetes, heart disease, or a thyroid gland disorder without a doctor's authorization.

POSSIBLE SIDE EFFECTS
Excessive doses of this product may result in nervousness, dizziness, or sleep disturbances. It also may interact with certain drugs prescribed for the treatment of depression or high blood pressure.

Amcill®

GENERIC NAME
Ampicillin.

PRODUCT CATEGORY
Broad-spectrum antibiotic (semisynthetic penicillin).

DOSAGE FORM
Liquid (oral suspension) and capsules.

WHY PRESCRIBED
Amcill is used to treat a wide range of bacterial infections in children, including those that involve the respiratory tract (breathing passages), digestive tract, and urinary tract.

CHILDREN'S DOSAGE
This depends largely on the type and severity of the infection and the child's age and weight. For infections of the respiratory tract, the usual dosage for children weighing less than 20 kilograms (44 pounds) is 50 milligrams per kilogram of body weight (1 kilogram = 2.2 pounds) each day, divided into equal-size doses given every six to eight hours. For children weighing more than 44 pounds, the usual dosage for respiratory infections is 250 milligrams every six hours. For infections of the digestive or urinary tracts, the usual dosage for children weighing less than 44 pounds is 100 milligrams per kilogram of body weight per day, given in equally divided doses every six to eight hours. The recommended dosage for treatment of digestive or urinary tract infections in children weighing more than 44 pounds is 500 milligrams every six hours.

PRECAUTIONS AND WARNINGS
Amcill should never be given to a child with a known allergic reaction to it or to penicillin. Adverse reactions are more likely if the child has experienced other allergies such as hay fever or hives (urticaria) or has asthma.

POSSIBLE SIDE EFFECTS
The most common side effects are diarrhea and skin rashes. Some children may also experience nausea and vomiting. More serious side effects are relatively uncommon.

amoxicillin (generic)

BRAND NAMES
Amoxil®, Augmentin®, Polymox®, Trimox®, Wymox®.

PRODUCT CATEGORY
Broad-spectrum antibiotic (semisynthetic penicillin).

DOSAGE FORM
Liquid (oral suspension), chewable tablets, and capsules.

WHY PRESCRIBED
Amoxicillin is used to treat a wide range of bacterial infections in children, including those that involve the ear, nose, and throat, urinary tract, skin, and lower part of the respiratory tract (air passages leading to the lungs).

CHILDREN'S DOSAGE
This depends largely on the type and severity of the infection and the child's age and weight. In general, the total dosage for infections of the skin, the urinary tract, or the ear, nose, and throat is 20 milligrams per kilogram of body weight (1 kilogram = 2.2 pounds) per day, given in divided doses every eight hours. Children who weigh more than 20 kilograms (44 pounds) should be given the adult dose of 250 milligrams every eight hours; that dosage may be doubled to 500 milligrams every eight hours for large children with certain severe infections of the lower air passages. The doctor also may advise giving larger doses to children weighing less than 44 pounds in cases of severe infections. Be sure to shake the bottle well before giving the oral suspension.

PRECAUTIONS AND WARNINGS
Amoxicillin should never be given to a child with a known allergic reaction to it or to penicillin. Adverse reactions are more likely if the child has experienced other allergies such as hay fever or hives (urticaria) or has asthma.

Long-term use of any antibiotic may result in the development of a "superinfection"—the growth and multiplication in the body of fungi of species of bacteria not affected by the medication. Dispose of any remaining amoxicillin once the course of therapy has been successfully completed.

POSSIBLE SIDE EFFECTS
Some children taking amoxicillin may experience diarrhea, nausea, vomiting, or skin rashes. More serious side effects are relatively uncommon.

Amoxil®

GENERIC NAME
Amoxicillin.

PRODUCT CATEGORY
Broad-spectrum antibiotic (semisynthetic penicillin).

DOSAGE FORM
Capsules, oral suspension, and chewable tablets.

WHY PRESCRIBED
Amoxil is used to treat a wide range of bacterial infections in children, including those that involve the ear, nose, and throat, urinary tract, skin, and lower part of the respiratory tract (air passages leading to the lungs).

CHILDREN'S DOSAGE
This depends largely on the type and severity of the infection and the child's age and weight. In general, the total daily dosage for infections of the skin, the urinary tract, or the ear, nose, and throat is 20 milligrams per kilogram of body weight (1 kilogram = 2.2 pounds), given in divided doses every eight hours. Children who weigh more than 20 kilograms (44 pounds) can be given the adult dose of 250 milligrams every eight hours. Larger doses may be prescribed by the doctor for severe infections. For infections of the lower part of the respiratory tract, the usual dosage is 40 milligrams per kilogram of body weight per day, given in divided doses every eight hours, and 500 milligrams every eight hours for children weighing more than 44 pounds. Be sure to shake the bottle well before giving the oral suspension.

PRECAUTIONS AND WARNINGS
Amoxil should never be given to a child with a known allergic reaction to it or to penicillin. Adverse reactions are more likely if the child has experienced other allergies such as hay fever or hives (urticaria) or has asthma.

Long-term use of any antibiotic may result in the development of a "superinfection"—the growth and multiplication in the body of fungi or of other species of bacteria not affected by the medication. Dispose of any remaining suspension or drops of Amoxil once the course of therapy has been successfully completed.

POSSIBLE SIDE EFFECTS
Some children taking Amoxil may experience diarrhea, nausea, vomiting, or skin rashes. More serious side effects are relatively uncommon.

ampicillin (generic)

BRAND NAMES
Amcill®, Omnipen®, Polycillin®, Principen®, SK-Ampicillin®, Totacillin®.

PRODUCT CATEGORY
Broad-spectrum antibiotic (semisynthetic penicillin).

DOSAGE FORM
Liquid (oral suspension); a capsule form is also available.

WHY PRESCRIBED
Ampicillin is used to treat a wide range of bacterial infections in children, including those that involve the middle ear (otitis media), stomach and intestines (gastrointestinal tract), urinary tract, the membranes that cover the brain (meningitis), and the skin.

CHILDREN'S DOSAGE
This depends largely on the severity of the infection and the child's age and weight. The site of the infection can also affect the dosage. For example, the usual dosage for children with an infection of the respiratory tract is 250 milligrams every six hours. However, if the child weighs less than 20 kilograms (44 pounds), the total daily dosage is usually 50 milligrams per kilogram of body weight (1 kilogram = 2.2 pounds), given in equally divided doses at intervals of six or eight hours. For pediatric suspension, follow specific instructions as the dosage also tends to vary with the size of the child and the type of infection. If it is kept refrigerated, ampicillin suspension remains stable for two weeks.

PRECAUTIONS AND WARNINGS
Ampicillin should never be given to a child with a known allergic reaction to it or to penicillin. Adverse reactions are more likely if the child has experienced other allergies such as hay fever or hives (urticaria). or has asthma

POSSIBLE SIDE EFFECTS
The most common side effects are diarrhea and skin rashes. Some children may also experience nausea and vomiting. More serious side effects are relatively uncommon.

Anacin® (OTC)

GENERIC NAME
This product contains a combination of **aspirin** (400 mg) and caffeine (32 mg).

PRODUCT CATEGORY
Analgesic/antipyretic/anti-inflammatory.

DOSAGE FORM
Tablets and capsules.

WHY USED
It is used to relieve pain (analgesic effect), reduce fever (antipyretic effect), and reduce redness and swelling (anti-inflammatory effect). Aspirin is useful in the symptomatic relief of headache, painful discomfort associated with the common cold and flu, muscular aches and pains, toothache, and various forms of arthritis.

CHILDREN'S DOSAGE
The usual recommended dosage for children between the ages of six and twelve is one tablet or capsule every four hours, as required. Do not give the child more than five tablets or capsules daily, unless otherwise advised by a doctor.

PRECAUTIONS AND WARNINGS
Children under the age of twelve should not take aspirin for more than five consecutive days or exceed the dosage on the label unless they are under medical supervision. Consult a physician immediately if pain persists in arthritic or rheumatic conditions affecting a child under twelve years of age.

Check with a doctor before giving aspirin to a child with bleeding problems (such as hemophilia), asthma, stomach problems, or allergies. Also, check with a doctor before giving an aspirin product to children, including teenagers, with chicken pox or flu.

To minimize irritation the stomach lining, give the child aspirin with food or a full glass of water.

Overdosage with aspirin can be fatal in young children.

POSSIBLE SIDE EFFECTS
The most common side effects include nausea, vomiting, and stomach pain. Children who are allergic to aspirin may occasionally experience itching, skin rash, shortness of breath, a tightness in the chest, and wheezing. Children who are allergic to aspirin can usually tolerate an OTC product that contains acetaminophen.

Aspirin may also cause minor bleeding from the stomach and intestinal tract.

ASPIRIN ALERT
Consult your doctor when giving aspirin products to reduce fever. The U.S. Department of Health and Human Services warns that giving aspirin to a child with fever increases the risk of Reye's syndrome. Read the notice on p. 15 ff.

Anacin-3® (OTC)
Acetaminophen for Children

GENERIC NAME
Acetaminophen.

PRODUCT CATEGORY
Analgesic/antipyretic.

DOSAGE FORM
Children's cherry-flavored chewable tablets (80 mg), cherry-flavored liquid (160 mg per 5 ml teaspoonful), fruit-flavored infant drops (80 mg per 0.8 ml dropperful).

WHY USED
It is used to reduce fever and relieve pain in upper respiratory infections such as the common cold and tonsillitis; headache; muscle ache (myalgia); the inflammation of the stomach or intestines (gastroenteritis); and reactions to vaccinations. It is also used to relieve pain and discomfort of many viral or bacterial infections such as earache (otitis media), sinus trouble, sore throat, and bronchitis.

CHILDREN'S DOSAGE
Dosages of Children's (80 mg) Anacin-3 chewable tablets depend upon the age and weight of the child according to the following recommended schedule:

Age of Child	Weight in Pounds	Tablets Every Four Hours
1–2 years	18–23	1½
2–3 years	24–35	2
4–5 years	36–47	3
6–8 years	48–59	4
9–10 years	60–71	5
11–12 years	72–95	6

Dosage of Anacin-3 liquid depends upon the age and weight of the child according to the following recommended schedule:

Age of Child	Weight	Teaspoonfuls Every Four Hours
4–11 months	12–17 pounds	½
12–23 months	18–23 pounds	¾
2–3 years	24–35 pounds	1
4–5 years	36–47 pounds	1½
6–8 years	48–59 pounds	2
9–10 years	60–71 pounds	2½
11–12 years	72–95 pounds	3

Anacin-3® (OTC)
Acetaminophen for Children (Continued)

Dosage of Infants' Anacin-3 Drops depends upon the age and weight of the child in the following recommended schedule:

Age of Child	Weight	Droppersful Every Four Hours
0–3 months	6–11 pounds	½
4–11 months	12–17 pounds	1
12–23 months	18–23 pounds	1½
2–3 years	24–35 pounds	2
4–5 years	36–47 pounds	3

PRECAUTIONS AND WARNINGS
Children should not be given more than five doses of acetaminophen in any five-hour period. Overdosage of acetaminophen may cause liver disorders in some children. Although such adverse reactions are rare, a doctor should be consulted in the event of any unusual signs or symptoms in a child who has taken acetaminophen. If a fever persists for more than three days or recurs, or if pain continues for more than five days while a child is taking acetaminophen, a doctor should be notified. Because the tablets contain an amino acid, phenylalanine, they should not be given to children with phenylketonuria (PKU) without a doctor's approval.

POSSIBLE SIDE EFFECTS
Acetaminophen is relatively free from side effects, making it useful for children who are allergic to aspirin. However, taking large doses or using the drug for a long period of time may result in itching, skin rashes, jaundice (yellowish coloring of the skin and whites of the eyes), and changes in the blood leading to a dangerous form of anemia.

Antepar®

GENERIC NAME
Piperazine.

PRODUCT CATEGORY
Antiparasitic.

DOSAGE FORM
Syrup and tablets (500 mg per tablet or teaspoonful).

WHY PRESCRIBED
It is used in the treatment of children with common roundworm infections (ascariasis) and pinworm infections (enterobiasis).

CHILDREN'S DOSAGE
This depends upon the weight of the child and the type of parasitic infection. The usual dosage is 75 milligrams per kilogram of body weight (1 kilogram = 2.2 pounds) in a single daily dose for two consecutive days. However, the total daily dose should not exceed 3.5 grams (seven tablets or seven teaspoonfuls) regardless of the weight of the child. Children with pinworm infections are usually given 65 milligrams per kilogram of body weight, administered as a single dose each day for seven consecutive days. The total daily dose should not exceed 2.5 grams (five tablets or five teaspoonfuls), regardless of the child's weight. In cases of severe infection, the course of treatment may have to be repeated after an interval of one week.

PRECAUTIONS AND WARNINGS
Antepar should not be given to children with epilepsy or other convulsive disorders or to those with impaired function of the kidneys or liver.

Prolonged treatment with this potentially toxic drug should be avoided. Do not give the child more than the prescribed dosage; this will minimize the possibility of adverse reactions.

POSSIBLE SIDE EFFECTS
Most of the reported side effects are related to giving the child more than the recommended dosage. These include nausea, vomiting, diarrhea, abdominal cramps, muscular incoordination, tremors, blurred vision, skin rashes, fever, joint pain, and various changes in behavior. Some children taking this drug may experience more serious side effects such as nerve disorders (neurotoxicity) and convulsions.

Stop giving the child Antepar at the first sign of an adverse reaction, and consult the physician immediately.

Antivert®

GENERIC NAME
Meclizine hydrochloride.

PRODUCT CATEGORY
Antiemetic (antihistamine).

DOSAGE FORM
Tablets in 12.5, 25, and 50 mg doses (a chewable tablet form is also available: 25 mg).

WHY PRESCRIBED
It is used to prevent or control the symptoms of motion sickness, including nausea, vomiting, and dizziness. Antivert is also possibly effective in the management of vertigo associated with disorders of the inner ear.

CHILDREN'S DOSAGE
Antivert should not be given to children under the age of twelve. For vertigo, the usual dosage for older children (and adults) is 25 to 100 milligrams daily, given in divided doses, depending on the needs and response of the child. For motion sickness, the recommended dosage is 25 to 50 milligrams taken one hour before the start of travel, with the same dose repeated every 24 hours for the remainder of the trip.

PRECAUTIONS AND WARNINGS
Antivert should not be given to a child with a known allergic reaction to the drug. It should be used only with a doctor's advice in cases of asthma, glaucoma, or other serious conditions.

POSSIBLE SIDE EFFECTS
The most commonly reported side effects are drowsiness, dryness of the mouth, and blurred vision.

aspirin (generic) (OTC)

BRAND NAMES
Examples of products for children that contain *only* aspirin include Bayer® Children's Chewable Aspirin and St. Joseph® Aspirin for Children. Many other products contain aspirin as one of the major ingredients (see *aspirin* in the Index at the back of this book).

Consult your doctor when giving aspirin products to reduce fever. The U.S. Department of Health and Human Services warns that giving aspirin to a child with fever increases the risk of Reye's syndrome. Read the notice on pp. 15 ff.

PRODUCT CATEGORY
Analgesic/antipyretic/anti-inflammatory.

DOSAGE FORM
Tablets, chewable tablets, and pediatric suppositories.

WHY USED
It is used to relieve pain (analgesic effect), reduce fever (antipyretic effect), and reduce redness and swelling (anti-inflammatory effect). Aspirin is useful in the relief of symptoms of headache, painful discomfort associated with the common cold and flu, muscular aches and pains, toothache, and various forms of arthritis.

In infants and very young children, aspirin is often used to prevent convulsions that might be caused by a high fever (fever-induced convulsions).

CHILDREN'S DOSAGE
Never give aspirin to children under the age of two years without the advice and supervision of a physician. Tablets or chewable tablets should usually be crushed and given with food or with milk, water, or other liquid to minimize the possibility of stomach irritation.

For the usual dosage of aspirin, see the entries for Bayer Children's Chewable Aspirin and St. Joseph Aspirin for Children. The suppository form of aspirin usually recommended by a physician. In such cases follow the prescribing instructions precisely or (if the child is not under medical care) follow the dosage instructions on the label.

Children should *never* be given adult doses of aspirin.

PRECAUTIONS AND WARNINGS
Children under the age of twelve should not take aspirin for more than five consecutive days or exceed the dosage on the label unless they are advised to do so by a physician.

Check with a physician before giving aspirin to a child with bleeding problems (such as hemophilia), asthma, stomach problems, or allergies.

Keep aspirin well out of the reach of small children. *An overdosage of aspirin can be fatal in the young.*

aspirin (generic) (OTC) (Continued)

Aspirin can reduce body temperature only when it is above normal. It has almost no effect on temperature in the absence of fever. Taken in the correct dosage, as recommended on the label, it usually provides effective relief within a few minutes. When it is taken in massive doses, however, it can actually *increase* the body temperature and cause a condition known as drug-induced fever.

Aspirin should not be used to reduce the fever and discomfort of chickenpox or influenza unless recommended by a physician.

POSSIBLE SIDE EFFECTS

The most common side effects include nausea, vomiting, and stomach pain. Children who are allergic to aspirin may occasionally experience itching, skin rash, shortness of breath, tightness in the chest, and wheezing. Children who are allergic to aspirin can usually tolerate an OTC product that contains the analgesic acetaminophen (for example, Children's Anacin-3®, Children's Panadol®, or Children's Tylenol®).

Excessive doses of aspirin can cause headache, visual disturbances, or ringing in the ears (tinnitus).

Aspirin may also cause minor bleeding from the stomach and intestines.

Atarax®

GENERIC NAME
Hydroxyzine hydrochloride.

PRODUCT CATEGORY
Sedative/minor tranquilizer/antiemetic.

DOSAGE FORM
Syrup and tablets.

WHY PRESCRIBED
Atarax is mainly used to help calm children who are emotionally disturbed, under stress, anxious, agitated, or apprehensive. The drug is also used to control nausea and vomiting (antiemetic action) and to relieve symptoms of allergies, particularly itching (pruritus) associated with skin conditions such as chronic urticaria (hives).

CHILDREN'S DOSAGE
The usual dosage for the control of anxiety and tension in children under the age of six years is 50 milligrams daily, given in divided doses. For children over the age of six, the dosage is between 50 and 100 milligrams daily, given in divided doses. The same dosages have been recommended for the relief of symptoms of urticaria and similar allergies in children. The physician should adjust the dosage depending on the severity of the condition being treated and the response of the child to Atarax therapy.

PRECAUTIONS AND WARNINGS
Do not give the child any other medicine at the same time as Atarax without a doctor's approval.

POSSIBLE SIDE EFFECTS
The most common side effect is drowsiness. Some children may also experience dryness of the mouth. Tremors and convulsions may result from giving greater than recommended doses of the product.

Augmentin®

GENERIC NAME
Amoxicillin with potassium clavulanate (an inhibitor of antibiotic-resistant organisms).

PRODUCT CATEGORY
Oral antibiotic.

DOSAGE FORM
Oral suspension, tablets, and chewable tablets.

WHY PRESCRIBED
It is used in the treatment of various bacterial infections, including those that involve the urinary tract, middle ear (otitis media), skin, sinuses (sinusitis), and lower respiratory tract (air passages leading to the lungs).

CHILDREN'S DOSAGE
The usual dose for infections of the middle ear, lower respiratory tract, and sinuses is 40 milligrams per kilogram of body weight (1 kilogram = 2.2 pounds) each day, given in divided doses every eight hours. For other infections, the recommended dosage is 20 milligrams per kilogram of body weight each day, given in divided doses every eight hours. Children who weigh more than 40 kilograms (88 pounds) should be given the adult dose of 250 milligrams every eight hours or 500 milligrams every eight hours in cases of severe infections.

PRECAUTIONS AND WARNINGS
Augmentin should not be given to any child known to be allergic to the product or to penicillin. Adverse reactions are more likely to occur in children who have experienced other allergies such as hay fever or hives (urticaria) or who have asthma.

Long-term use of any antibiotic may result in the development of a "superinfection"—the growth and multiplication in the body of fungi or of species of bacteria not affected by the medication. Dispose of any remaining supplies of the product once the course of therapy has been successfully completed.

POSSIBLE SIDE EFFECTS
Some children taking amoxicillin products may experience diarrhea, nausea, vomiting, or skin rashes. More serious side effects are relatively uncommon.

Auralgan® Otic Solution

GENERIC NAME
This product contains the following combination of ingredients in each milliliter: antipyrine (54 mg), benzocaine (14 mg), and dehydrated glycerin (1 ml).

PRODUCT CATEGORY
Otic (ear) preparation.

DOSAGE FORM
Solution (for instillation directly into the outer ear canal).

WHY PRESCRIBED
It is used to relieve the symptoms of infections of the middle ear (acute otitis media), including pain and inflammation. Auralgan also helps loosen hardened earwax (impacted cerumen).

CHILDREN'S DOSAGE
The prescribing physician will give detailed instructions for the use of this product.

PRECAUTIONS AND WARNINGS
Children who are hypersensitive (allergic) to any of the ingredients of Auralgan should not be given this drug.

Children with a perforated eardrum or discharge from the ear should not use Auralgan. In such cases, consult the doctor at once.

POSSIBLE SIDE EFFECTS
No significant side effects have been reported.

Azo Gantrisin®

GENERIC NAME
This product contains a combination of sulfisoxazole and phenazopyridine hydrochloride.

PRODUCT CATEGORY
Antibacterial (sulfonamide) and urinary analgesic.

DOSAGE FORM
Tablets.

WHY PRESCRIBED
It is used mainly in children over the age of twelve (as well as adults) to treat bacterial infections of the kidneys and bladder during the acute early stages of the infection. Azo Gantrisin also relieves the pain and burning sensation that often accompanies such infections.

CHILDREN'S DOSAGE
This drug should not be used to treat children under the age of twelve. The usual dosage for older children (and adults) is two tablets four times daily for no more than two days. Treatment beyond the first two days should be with another sulfonamide product (Gantrisin®).

PRECAUTIONS AND WARNINGS
If the painful symptoms of infection of the urinary tract do not improve during the treatment period, consult your doctor at once. The bacteria responsible may have become resistant to the effects of Azo Gantrisin, and another drug may be required to cure the condition.

Have the child drink plenty of water while taking this drug to help prevent the formation of crystals of Azo Gantrisin in the kidneys.

POSSIBLE SIDE EFFECTS
The most common side effects experienced by some children taking Azo Gantrisin include headache, nausea, vomiting, diarrhea, stomach pain or discomfort, and a sensation of ringing in the ears (tinnitus). Drugs in this class (the sulfa drugs) may also cause potentially serious allergic reactions in some children.

One of the ingredients in Azo Gantrisin (phenazopyridine hydrochloride) causes the urine to turn orange-red. Be sure to tell the child that this is *absolutely harmless* and disappears once therapy has been completed.

Baby Anbesol® (OTC)

GENERIC NAME
The product is a combination of benzocaine (7.5 percent), Carbomer 934, D&C Red No. 33, disodium edetate, glycerin, polyethylene glycol, saccharin, and water.

PRODUCT CATEGORY
Topical (local) anesthetic.

DOSAGE FORM
Clear gel.

WHY USED
It is used to provide quick, temporary relief from the pain and discomfort experienced by infants during teething. The product blocks painful nerve impulses from the sore gum tissues.

CHILDREN'S DOSAGE
A small amount of the gel is applied to the child's gums with a cotton swab or the fingertip.

PRECAUTIONS AND WARNINGS
If teething pain is persistent or excessive, a doctor should be consulted. The product should be handled only by adults. It should not get into the eyes or onto the skin around the eyes. Children are more likely to be sensitive to skin absorption and adverse reactions from contact with substances containing topical anesthetics such as benzocaine.

POSSIBLE SIDE EFFECTS
Baby Anbesol is relatively free from serious side effects when used according to instructions. Itching, skin rashes, and nervous system disorders are among the infrequent side effects of topical anesthetics.

Bactrim®

GENERIC NAME
This product contains trimethoprim and sulfamethoxazole.

PRODUCT CATEGORY
Antibacterial (combination including a sulfonamide).

DOSAGE FORM
Liquid (oral suspension), containing in each teaspoonful (5 ml) 40 mg of trimethoprim and 200 mg of sulfamethoxazole, and tablets, containing 80 mg of trimethoprim and 400 mg of sulfamethoxazole.

WHY PRESCRIBED
It is mainly used in children to treat bacterial infections of the urinary tract (kidneys and bladder) and those that involve the middle ear (acute otitis media).

CHILDREN'S DOSAGE

Weight of Child	Tablets	Teaspoonfuls (5 ml) Every 12 Hours
22 lb (10 kg)	½	1
44 lb (20 kg)	1	2
66 lb (30 kg)	1½	3
88 lb (40 kg)	2	4

PRECAUTIONS AND WARNINGS
Stop giving Bactrim to a child who develops a skin rash, sore throat, or yellowness of the skin, and consult a physician immediately.

Have the child drink plenty of water while taking Bactrim to help prevent the formation of crystals in the kidneys.

Bactrim should not be given to infants under the age of two months.

Bactrim should never be used to treat a strep throat.

Before giving the child this drug, be sure the physician is aware of any history of severe allergies, bronchial asthma, or problems with the child's kidneys or liver.

POSSIBLE SIDE EFFECTS
The most common side effects experienced by some children taking Bactrim include headache, nausea, vomiting, diarrhea, stomach pain or discomfort, and ringing in the ears (tinnitus).

Bactrim contains a sulfa drug (sulfamethoxazole), which may cause a potentially serious allergic reaction in some children.

Bayer® Children's Chewable Aspirin (OTC)

GENERIC NAME
Aspirin (81 mg).

PRODUCT CATEGORY
Analgesic/antipyretic/anti-inflammatory.

DOSAGE FORM
Chewable tablets (orange flavor).

WHY USED
It is used to relieve pain (analgesic effect), reduce fever (antipyretic effect), and reduce redness and swelling (anti-inflammatory effect). Aspirin is useful in the symptomatic relief of headache, painful discomfort associated with the common cold, muscular aches and pains, toothache, and various forms of arthritis.

CHILDREN'S DOSAGE
Do not give this product to children under the age of three without the advice and supervision of a physician. Consult a doctor before giving aspirin to any child, including teenagers, with chickenpox or flu.

Age of Child	Tablets Every 4 Hours if Needed
3–under 4 years	2
4–under 6 years	3
6–under 9 years	4
9–under 11 years	5
11–under 12 years	6

Do not give a child the recommended dosage more than five times a day. Larger doses may be prescribed by a physician. Give the tablets with food or with milk, water, or other liquid to minimize the possibility of stomach upset.

PRECAUTIONS AND WARNINGS
Children under the age of twelve should not take aspirin for more than five consecutive days or exceed the dosage on the label unless they do so under medical supervision.

Check with a physician before giving aspirin to a child with bleeding problems (such as hemophilia), asthma, stomach problems, or allergies.
Overdosage with aspirin can be fatal in young children.

Bayer® Children's Chewable Aspirin (OTC) (Continued)

POSSIBLE SIDE EFFECTS

The most common side effects include nausea, vomiting, and stomach pain. Children who are allergic to aspirin may occasionally experience itching, skin rash, shortness of breath, a tightness in the chest, and wheezing. Children who are allergic to aspirin can usually tolerate an OTC product that contains acetaminophen (such as Children's Anacin-3®, Children's Panadol®, or Children's Tylenol®).

Aspirin may also cause minor bleeding from the stomach and intestines.

ASPIRIN ALERT
Consult your doctor when giving aspirin products to reduce fever. The U.S. Department of Health and Human Services warns that giving aspirin to a child with fever increases the risk of Reye's syndrome. Read the notice on pp. 15 ff.

Bayer® Children's Cold Tablets (OTC)

GENERIC NAME
This product contains a combination of phenylpropanolamine hydrochloride (3.125 mg) and **aspirin** (81 mg).

PRODUCT CATEGORY
Decongestant/analgesic (pain reliever).

DOSAGE FORM
Tablets.

WHY USED
It is used to relieve the symptoms of the common cold or flu, including stuffy nose (nasal congestion), fever, and minor discomfort.

CHILDREN'S DOSAGE
Bayer Children's Cold Tablets are available without a doctor's prescription. Administer to children exactly as the label recommends.

PRECAUTIONS AND WARNINGS
Unless you are so advised by a physician, do not give this drug to children with heart disorders, diabetes, asthma, high blood pressure, or thyroid disease.

POSSIBLE SIDE EFFECTS
Some children taking this product may experience nervousness, dizziness, or insomnia.

ASPIRIN ALERT
Consult your doctor when giving aspirin products to reduce fever. The U.S. Department of Health and Human Services warns that giving aspirin to a child with fever increases the risk of Reye's syndrome. Read the notice on pp. 15 ff.

Benadryl® (OTC)

GENERIC NAME
Diphenhydramine hydrochloride.

PRODUCT CATEGORY
Antihistamine.

DOSAGE FORM
Capsules (25 mg).

WHY USED
It is used mainly to relieve the symptoms of allergies such as hay fever (allergic rhinitis), hives (urticaria), and allergic conjunctivitis. It is also effective in preventing or relieving the symptoms of motion sickness.

CHILDREN'S DOSAGE
The usual dosage for children who weigh over 20 pounds is 12.5 to 25 milligrams three or four times a day, and a daily total of not more than 300 milligrams. The manufacturer recommends that the prescribing physician adjust the dosage according to the needs and the response of the child.

PRECAUTIONS AND WARNINGS
Benadryl should not be given to newborn or premature infants or used to treat children who have asthma or other disorders of the lower respiratory tract. Do not give Benadryl to children who are hypersensitive (allergic) to antihistamines.

POSSIBLE SIDE EFFECTS
The most commonly reported side effects include sedation, drowsiness, disturbed coordination, dizziness, and a thickening of the secretions in the lower air passages (bronchial tubes). The nose, mouth, and throat may also become excessively dry.

Benadryl is an antihistamine. In infants and children, an overdosage of antihistamine may cause hallucinations, convulsions, or even death.

Bentyl®

GENERIC NAME
Dicyclomine hydrochloride.

PRODUCT CATEGORY
Antispasmodic.

DOSAGE FORM
Syrup and capsules (a tablet form is also available).

WHY PRESCRIBED
It is used to relieve muscular spasms of the stomach and intestines associated with various diseases and disorders of the gastrointestinal tract.

CHILDREN'S DOSAGE
The physician will adjust the dosage according to the needs of the individual child and the severity of the symptoms. The usual dosage for children is one capsule or one teaspoonful (5 ml) of syrup, given three or four times daily. It should not be given to infants under the age of six months; older infants are usually given one-half teaspoonful (2.5 ml) of syrup diluted with an equal amount of water, administered three or four times daily.

PRECAUTIONS AND WARNINGS
Bentyl should be used with caution in children with heart disorders, thyroid disease, or impaired function of the kidneys or liver.

POSSIBLE SIDE EFFECTS
These include nervousness, drowsiness, headache, blurred vision, loss of taste, difficulty urinating, increase in heart rate (tachycardia), sensation of heartbeat (palpitations), dizziness, nausea, vomiting, constipation, drug-induced skin rashes, and (rarely) a severe generalized allergic reaction (anaphylactic shock).

Benylin® Cough Syrup (OTC)

GENERIC NAME
This product contains in each teaspoonful (5 ml) a combination of diphenhydramine hydrochloride (12.5 mg), alcohol (5 percent), and various other ingredients, including flavorings and colorings.

PRODUCT CATEGORY
Antitussive (cough suppressant)/antihistamine.

DOSAGE FORM
Syrup.

WHY USED
It is used to relieve coughing associated with inhaled irritants or the common cold.

CHILDREN'S DOSAGE
Benylin Cough Syrup should not be given to children under the age of six years without the approval of the doctor. The usual dosage for children between the ages of six and twelve years is one teaspoonful (5 ml) every four hours. Do not give the child more than six teaspoonfuls in any 24-hour period, unless advised by a physician. The prescribing physician should recommend the dosage for a child between the ages of two and six and decide if the product should be given at all to a child under the age of two.

PRECAUTIONS AND WARNINGS
Benylin Cough Syrup should not be given to a child with asthma, a persistent cough, a cough accompanied by excessive secretions, or certain other conditions, such as epilepsy, without the advice and supervision of a doctor.

Benylin Cough Syrup contains a potent antihistamine (diphenhydramine hydrochloride). In children, an overdosage of antihistamine may cause hallucinations, convulsions, or even death.

POSSIBLE SIDE EFFECTS
The most commonly reported side effects include sedation, dizziness, impaired coordination, drowsiness, abdominal discomfort, and thickening of the secretions in the lower air passages (bronchial tubes). Less commonly, a child may experience dryness of the mouth, nose, and throat; drug-induced skin rash; headache; increased heartrate (tachycardia); sensation of heartbeat (palpitations);
blurred vision; ringing in the ears (tinnitus); extreme excitability; nausea; vomiting; tightness in the chest; wheezing; and difficulty urinating.

A few patients using this product have experienced a severe allergic reaction (anaphylactic shock) or serious impairment of the blood-forming tissues.

Benylin DM® Cough Syrup

GENERIC NAME
This product contains in each teaspoonful (5 ml) a combination of dextromethorphan (10 mg), alcohol (5 percent), and various other ingredients, including flavorings and colorings.

PRODUCT CATEGORY
Antitussive (cough suppressant).

DOSAGE FORM
Syrup (raspberry flavor).

WHY PRESCRIBED
It is used for temporary relief of coughing associated with minor throat and bronchial irritation.

CHILDREN'S DOSAGE
Benylin DM should not be given to children under the age of two years without the advice and supervision of a doctor. For children two to six years old, the recommended dosage is ¼ to ½ teaspoonful every four hours, or ¾ teaspoonful every six to eight hours. The recommended dosage for children between two and six years is three teaspoonfuls in 24 hours. For children between six and twelve years of age, the recommended dosage is ½ to 1 teaspoonful every four hours, or 1 teaspoonful every six to eight hours, with a maximum daily total of six teaspoonfuls.

PRECAUTIONS AND WARNINGS
Benylin DM should not be given to a child with a liver disorder, asthma, or a chronic or persistent cough, or a cough accompanied by excessive secretions, except with the advice and supervision of a doctor. If the cough persists for more than a week or is accompanied by a fever or headache, consult a doctor. If the child is allergic to any cough syrup or to dextromethorphan, consult a doctor.

POSSIBLE SIDE EFFECTS
Few serious side effects have been reported with this product, the exceptions being rare occurrences of dizziness or drowsiness, skin rashes, and digestive upsets. If adverse effects are observed, it is recommended that use of the product be discontinued until a doctor is consulted.

Bonine® (OTC)

GENERIC NAME
Meclizine hydrochloride.

PRODUCT CATEGORY
Antiemetic (antihistamine).

DOSAGE FORM
Chewable tablets (25 mg).

WHY USED
It is used for the prevention or control of the symptoms of motion sickness, including nausea, vomiting, and dizziness.

CHILDREN'S DOSAGE
Bonine is available without a doctor's prescription. Administer to children exactly as the label recommends. This drug is not recommended for children under the age of twelve. For motion sickness, the usual dose is one or two tablets taken one hour before the start of travel, with an additional one or two tablets during each 24 hours that the trip continues.

PRECAUTIONS AND WARNINGS
Bonine should not be given to a child with a known allergic reaction to this product or to similar drugs. A doctor should be consulted before giving the drug to a child with asthma or any other chronic disorder.

POSSIBLE SIDE EFFECTS
The most commonly reported side effects are drowsiness, dryness of the mouth, and blurred vision.

Bronitin® Tablets (OTC)

GENERIC NAME
This product contains a combination of ephedrine hydrochloride (24 mg), pyrilamine maleate (16.6 mg), theophylline (120 mg), and guaifenesin (100 mg).

PRODUCT CATEGORY
Brochodilator/antiasthmatic/expectorant.

DOSAGE FORM
Tablets.

WHY USED
It helps relieve wheezing and shortness of breath in children with bronchial asthma. It is also designed to loosen phlegm and mucus in the air passages (expectorant action).

CHILDREN'S DOSAGE
Bronitin is available without a doctor's prescription. It should be administered to children exactly as the label recommends.

PRECAUTIONS AND WARNINGS
Do not give a child Bronitin unless a medical diagnosis of asthma has been made. Do not give this product to children with a heart disorder, high blood pressure (hypertension), or diabetes without approval by a physician.

Children with symptoms of asthma should be examined by a physician. The best treatment often involves the use of more effective prescription drugs.

If the child's symptoms fail to improve, seek medical attention at once.

POSSIBLE SIDE EFFECTS
Some children may experience nervousness, restlessness, and sleeplessness. Should any of these side effects occur, stop giving the child Bronitin and consult a doctor.

The antihistamine ingredient in Bronitin (pyrilamine maleate) can cause drowsiness. Excessive amounts of antihistamine in children can cause potentially serious side effects.

Bronitin® Mist (OTC)

GENERIC NAME
Epinephrine (as bitartrate 0.5 percent).

PRODUCT CATEGORY
Bronchodilator/antiasthmatic.

DOSAGE FORM
Aerosol (to be inhaled).

WHY USED
It helps relieve wheezing and shortness of breath in children with bronchial asthma.

CHILDREN'S DOSAGE
Bronitin Mist is available without a doctor's prescription. If prompt relief is not obtained after following the directions on the label (usually one or two applications), consult a physician.

PRECAUTIONS AND WARNINGS
Do not give a child Bronitin Mist unless a medical diagnosis of asthma has been made. Overuse of aerosol bronchodilators can be dangerous. Medical supervision of asthma, especially in children, is extremely important.

POSSIBLE SIDE EFFECTS
Serious side effects are uncommon. However, overdependence on treatment that is not effective may permit the condition to progress to a point where it becomes a direct threat to life.

If the child's symptoms fail to improve, consult a doctor.

Bronkaid® Mist and Mist Suspension (OTC)

GENERIC NAME
Epinephrine (0.5 percent in mist; as bitartrate 0.5 percent in mist suspension).

PRODUCT CATEGORY
Bronchodilator/anti-asthmatic

DOSAGE FORM
Aerosol (to be inhaled).

WHY USED
It helps relieve wheezing and shortness of breath in children with bronchial asthma.

CHILDREN'S DOSAGE
Bronkaid Mist is available without a doctor's prescription. If prompt relief is not obtained after following the directions on the label (usually one or two applications), consult a physician.

PRECAUTIONS AND WARNINGS
Do not give a child Bronkaid Mist unless a medical diagnosis of asthma has been made. Overuse of aerosol bronchodilators can be dangerous. Medical supervision of asthma, especially in children, is extremely important.

POSSIBLE SIDE EFFECTS
Serious side effects are uncommon. However, overdependence on treatment that is not effective may permit the condition to progress to a point where it becomes a direct threat to life.

If the child's symptoms fail to improve, consult a doctor.

Bronkaid® Tablets (OTC)

GENERIC NAME
This product contains a combination of ephedrine sulfate (24 mg), theophylline (100 mg), and guaifenesin (100 mg).

PRODUCT CATEGORY
Bronchodilator/antiasthmatic/expectorant.

DOSAGE FORM
Tablets.

WHY USED
It helps relieve wheezing and shortness of breath in children with bronchial asthma and loosens phlegm and mucus.

CHILDREN'S DOSAGE
Bronkaid Tablets are available without a doctor's prescription. Administer to children exactly as the label recommends. Tablets should be swallowed whole with water.

PRECAUTIONS AND WARNINGS
Do not give a child Bronkaid Tablets unless a diagnosis of asthma has been made by a physician. Do not give this product to children with a heart disorder, thyroid disease, high blood pressure (hypertension), diabetes, or persistent cough without approval by a physician.

Children with asthma should be examined by a doctor. The best treatment often involves the use of more effective prescription drugs.

If the child's symptoms fail to improve, seek medical attention at once.

POSSIBLE SIDE EFFECTS
The most commonly reported side effects include nervousness, restlessness, and sleeplessness. Some children may also experience difficulty urinating. Should any of these side effects occur, stop giving the child Bronkaid and consult a physician.

Bronkotabs® (OTC)

GENERIC NAME
This product contains a combination of ephedrine sulfate (24 mg), theophylline (100 mg), phenobarbital (8 mg), and guaifenesin (100 mg).

PRODUCT CATEGORY
Bronchodilator/antiasthmatic/expectorant.

DOSAGE FORM
Tablets.

WHY USED
It helps relieve wheezing and shortness of breath in children with bronchial asthma. It is also designed to loosen phlegm and mucus in the air passages (expectorant action).

CHILDREN'S DOSAGE
In some states, Bronkotabs may be available only with a doctor's prescription (because the phenobarbital ingredient can be habit-forming). In such cases the physician will determine the appropriate dosage for each child. Severe forms of asthma will require more effective prescription drugs to control attacks. In areas where the drug may be available without a prescription, administer to the child exactly as the label recommends.

PRECAUTIONS AND WARNINGS
Do not give a child Bronkotabs unless a medical diagnosis of asthma has been made. Do not give the product to a child with a heart disorder, high blood pressure (hypertension), diabetes, thyroid disease, or persistent cough unless you are directed to do so by a physician.

Children with symptoms of asthma should be examined by a physician. The best treatment often involves the use of more effective prescription drugs.

If the child's condition fails to improve, seek medical attention at once.

POSSIBLE SIDE EFFECTS
Some children may experience nervousness, restlessness, or sleeplessness. Should any of these effects occur, stop giving the child Bronkotabs and consult a physician.

The phenobarbital ingredient in this product can be habit-forming, especially if it is taken in excessive amounts for prolonged periods.

Butisol Sodium®

GENERIC NAME
Sodium butabarbital.

PRODUCT CATEGORY
Sedative/hypnotic (sleep-inducing drug).

DOSAGE FORM
Elixir (liquid containing 30 mg per 5 ml teaspoonful) and tablets.

WHY PRESCRIBED
It is used as a daytime sedative for children to help calm anxiety or other emotional disturbances or to help induce sleep at bedtime.

CHILDREN'S DOSAGE
This depends on the severity of symptoms and the age and weight of the child. The physician will prescribe the specific dosage, depending on the needs and response of the individual child.

PRECAUTIONS AND WARNINGS
This drug should not be given to children who are sensitive to barbiturates. It also should not be given to children with an inborn (hereditary) error of metabolism known as porphyria.

The prolonged use of Butisol Sodium may lead to drug dependence and to severe withdrawal symptoms if its use is abruptly discontinued.

POSSIBLE SIDE EFFECTS
Among the reported side effects of this class of drug are respiratory depression, nausea, vomiting, skin rashes, lethargy, and residual sedation ("drug hangover").

Caladryl® (OTC)

GENERIC NAME
This product contains a combination of Benadryl® (diphenhydramine hydrochloride), calamine, and camphor.

PRODUCT CATEGORY
Topical drying agent/antihistamine.

DOSAGE FORM
Cream and lotion.

WHY USED
It is used to relieve itching and minor irritation of the skin associated with insect bites, mild sunburn, or contact with poison ivy, poison oak, or poison sumac.

CHILDREN'S DOSAGE
Caladryl is available without a doctor's prescription. Administer to children exactly as the label recommends, carefully cleansing the skin with soap and water and drying the area before applying the cream or lotion.

PRECAUTIONS AND WARNINGS
Caladryl should not be applied to skin areas that are blistered, oozing, or raw. It also should not be used around the eyes or other mucous membranes (such as the mouth or nostrils).

Do not use the product for more than seven days or on large areas of the skin without the advice of a physician.

Caladryl is for use only on irritated skin areas.

POSSIBLE SIDE EFFECTS
Some children may experience a burning sensation or skin rash from use of the product. If this occurs, remove the cream or lotion with soap and water and discontinue its use.

The camphor and diphenhydramine in Caladryl can cause serious toxicity, including seizures, if the product is swallowed.

Calcidrine® Syrup

GENERIC NAME
This product contains a combination of codeine (8.4 mg), calcium iodide (152 mg), alcohol (6 percent), and various inactive ingredients such as flavorings and colorings.

PRODUCT CATEGORY
Antitussive (cough suppressant)/expectorant.

DOSAGE FORM
Syrup.

WHY PRESCRIBED
It is used to relieve the symptoms of coughs and to help loosen phlegm and mucus in the air passages (expectorant **action).**

CHILDREN'S DOSAGE

Age of Child	Teaspoonfuls (5 ml) Every 4 Hours
2–6 years	½
6–10 years	½–1
Over 10 years	1–2

PRECAUTIONS AND WARNINGS
Calcidrine Syrup contains codeine, which may be habit forming and, in the event of accidental overdosage, can depress the child's breathing and nervous system functions. It should not be given to a child who is known to be hypersensitive (allergic) to iodides (iodine compounds). The prescribing physician should be consulted about any health condition of the child, including the use of other medications at the same time, that may be affected by use of the product.

POSSIBLE SIDE EFFECTS
Side effects that have been reported include acne or other skin eruptions, a metallic taste, irritation of the mucous membranes, swollen salivary glands, and gastrointestinal (digestive tract) upsets. Some children may experience nausea, vomiting, or constipation because of the presence of codeine in the product. The side effects usually disappear when use of the drug is discontinued.

CaldeCORT® (OTC)

GENERIC NAME
Hydrocortisone acetate.

PRODUCT CATEGORY
Anti-inflammatory (corticosteroid).

DOSAGE FORM
Cream and aerosol spray.

WHY USED
CaldeCORT relieves the itching and discomfort of minor skin irritations resulting from poison ivy, poison oak, poison sumac, insect bites, and allergic skin reactions to certain household products such as soaps and detergents.

CHILDREN'S DOSAGE
CaldeCORT should not be applied to the skin of children under the age of two without the advice and supervision of a physician. For children two years of age and older, the cream or spray may be applied to the affected area three or four times a day.

PRECAUTIONS AND WARNINGS
This product is for use only on irritated areas of the skin. It should not be applied around the eyes or other mucous membranes (such as the mouth or nostrils). The product should not be used for more than seven days without the approval of a doctor. A physician should be consulted if the symptoms worsen during use of the product.

POSSIBLE SIDE EFFECTS
The most commonly reported side effects of hydrocortisone products include skin eruptions, thirst, and digestive system disorders, such as nausea and vomiting. Less common effects are blurred vision, muscle cramps, and fever.

Ceclor®

GENERIC NAME
Cefaclor.

PRODUCT CATEGORY
Antibiotic (semisynthetic cephalosporin).

DOSAGE FORM
Liquid (oral suspension) and capsules.

WHY PRESCRIBED
It is used to treat certain bacterial infections, such as those that involve the middle ear (otitis media), the upper part of the respiratory tract (tonsillitis and sore throat), and the urinary tract (kidneys and bladder).

CHILDREN'S DOSAGE
The usual total daily dosage for children is 20 milligrams per kilogram of body weight (1 kilogram = 2.2 pounds), given in divided doses every eight hours. In treating particularly severe infections, such as those involving the middle ear, the prescribing doctor may increase this amount. The maximum total dosage should not exceed 1 gram (four 5 ml teaspoonfuls of the 250 mg oral suspension). Ceclor is not recommended for infants less than one month old or weighing less than 20 pounds.

PRECAUTIONS AND WARNINGS
Some children who are allergic to penicillin may also be allergic to Ceclor. In such cases, the drug must be used with great caution (if at all). If symptoms of an allergic reaction are observed, discontinue use of the drug. Prolonged use of the drug may lead to development of a "superinfection"—an overgrowth of disease organisms that are resistant to Ceclor. Oral suspensions of Ceclor should be kept in a refrigerator and any unused portion discarded after 14 days.

POSSIBLE SIDE EFFECTS
The most common side effects are diarrhea, nausea, vomiting, itching, and hives (urticaria).

Cerumenex® Drops

GENERIC NAME
Triethanolamine polypeptide oleate-condensate (10 percent) with 0.5 percent chlorobutanol in propylene gycol.

PRODUCT CATEGORY
Cerumenolytic/otic (ear) preparation.

DOSAGE FORM
Solution (for instillation directly into the outer ear canal).

WHY PRESCRIBED
It is used to emulsify and disperse impacted or excessive earwax (cerumen) so it can be removed without the use of instruments.

CHILDREN'S DOSAGE
The physician will give detailed instructions on the use of this product.

PRECAUTIONS AND WARNINGS
Cerumenex should be used with extreme caution (if at all) in children with allergies.

Do not leave drops of Cerumenex in the outer ear canal for more than 15 to 30 minutes or exceed the frequency of use recommended by the child's physician.

Children with a perforated eardrum or discharge from the ear should not use Cerumenex. In such cases, consult the doctor at once.

POSSIBLE SIDE EFFECTS
Some children may experience allergic skin reactions. Should this occur, stop using the drug and consult the physician.

Children's Chloraseptic® Lozenges (OTC)

GENERIC NAME
Benzocaine (5 mg).

PRODUCT CATEGORY
Topical (local) anesthetic.

DOSAGE FORM
Lozenge (grape flavor).

WHY USED
It is used to provide temporary relief of minor sore throat pain that may accompany inflammation of the tonsils or throat, soreness following a tonsillectomy, or irritation of the mouth and gums.

CHILDREN'S DOSAGE
Chloraseptic Lozenges are available without a doctor's prescription. If prompt relief is not obtained after following the directions on the label, consult a physician. The product is not recommended for children under the age of five years without the advice of a physician or dentist.

PRECAUTIONS AND WARNINGS
A sore throat may be a symptom of a serious disease. If the condition is severe or lasts more than two days or is accompanied by a fever, headache, nausea, or vomiting, a doctor should be consulted.

POSSIBLE SIDE EFFECTS
Serious side effects from the use of products containing benzocaine are uncommon but may include dizziness, skin rash, blurred vision, slow heartbeat, and swelling of the feet.

Chloromycetin®

GENERIC NAME
Chloramphenicol.

PRODUCT CATEGORY
Antibiotic.

DOSAGE FORM
Liquid (oral suspension) and capsules (other forms are also available, including ear drops, topical cream, and ophthalmic ointment).

WHY PRESCRIBED
This extremely potent antibiotic should be used only to treat potentially life-threatening infections or when the invading microorganisms fail to respond to other antibiotics that pose a reduced risk of serious side effects. Chloromycetin is mainly used to treat typhoid fever, severe cases of meningitis (inflammation of the membranes that cover the brain and spinal cord), and Rocky Mountain spotted fever.

CHILDREN'S DOSAGE
The usual dosage for children is 50 milligrams per kilogram of body weight (1 kilogram = 2.2 pounds) per day, divided into four doses given at intervals of six hours.

PRECAUTIONS AND WARNINGS
Chloromycetin must never be used to treat trivial infections or to prevent infections. Many physicians recommend that the drug be administered to children only if they are under direct medical supervision in a hospital. This makes it easier to follow the progress of the child and to perform the essential blood tests that are required during treatment.

POSSIBLE SIDE EFFECTS
Chloramphenicol (the active ingredient of Chloromycetin) is one of the most toxic antibiotics available. Used properly, it can be lifesaving. However, in a few patients it can cause potentially fatal side effects, including aplastic anemia and other disorders of the blood-forming tissues.

Chloroptic® S.O.P. Opthalmic

GENERIC NAME
This product contains a combination of chloramphenicol (1 percent) and chlorobutanol (0.5 percent).

PRODUCT CATEGORY
Ophthalmic anti-infective/anesthetic.

DOSAGE FORM
Sterile ophthalmic ointment.

WHY PRESCRIBED
It is used to treat susceptible bacterial infections of the eye (conjunctiva or cornea).

CHILDREN'S DOSAGE
This depends largely on the severity of the infection and the child's response to Chloroptic therapy. The physician will determine the appropriate individual dosage.

PRECAUTIONS AND WARNING
This drug is not intended for long-term use. If no improvement is seen within three days, consult the doctor.

Stop using the drug and notify the doctor if the child shows signs of an allergic reaction, such as constant burning or itching of the eyelids.

POSSIBLE SIDE EFFECTS
The most common side effects are a stinging or burning sensation after the drug is applied. Some children may be allergic to Chloroptic, resulting in itching or burning of the eye or signs of inflammation of the eyelid. Prolonged use of Chloroptic may pose the risk of more serious side effects, including impairment of the blood-forming tissues.

Chlor-Trimeton® Allergy Syrup (OTC)

GENERIC NAME
Chlorpheniramine maleate (2 mg per 5 ml teaspoonful) and alcohol (7 percent).

PRODUCT CATEGORY
Antihistamine.

DOSAGE FORM
Syrup and tablets.

WHY USED
It is used to relieve the symptoms of hay fever and other allergies that affect the upper part of the respiratory tract.

CHILDREN'S DOSAGE
Chlor-Trimeton Allergy Syrup is available without a doctor's prescription. Administer to children exactly as the label recommends.

PRECAUTIONS AND WARNINGS
Unless advised by a physician, do not give this drug to children under the age of six or to those with asthma.

POSSIBLE SIDE EFFECTS
The most common side effect is drowsiness. Chlor-Trimetron contains an antihistamine (chlorpheniramine maleate). In infants and children overdosage of antihistamine may cause hallucinations, convulsions, or even death.

Cleocin Pediatric®

GENERIC NAME
Clindamycin palmitate hydrochloride.

PRODUCT CATEGORY
Antibiotic.

DOSAGE FORM
Liquid (flavored granules reconstituted with water).

WHY PRESCRIBED
It is used in the treatment of a wide range of severe bacterial infections, including susceptible strains of streptococci, pneumococci, and staphylococci. The drug is also used to treat infections caused by certain types of anaerobic bacteria (those that thrive in the absence of oxygen). Physicians generally restrict the use of Cleocin to children who are allergic to penicillin, which might otherwise be the drug of choice.

CHILDREN'S DOSAGE
This depends largely on the severity of the infection and the child's weight. The usual dosage ranges from 4 to 6 milligrams per pound of body weight per day, divided into three or four equal doses, for serious infections and ranging upward to between 17 and 25 milligrams per kilogram (or 8.5 to 12.5 milligrams per pound) of body weight per day, divided into three or four equal doses, for very severe infections. (Each 5 ml teaspoonful of reconstituted Cleocin Pediatric contains the equivalent of 75 mg of the drug.)

PRECAUTIONS AND WARNINGS
Cleocin Pediatric should be used with extreme caution in children with a disease or disorder of the gastrointestinal tract (stomach and intestines), especially those with colitis.

If the child experiences significant diarrhea while taking Cleocin, discontinue the use of the drug and consult a physician.

Do *not* refrigerate this drug as it may become thick and difficult to pour. Cleocin remains stable at room temperature for two weeks.

POSSIBLE SIDE EFFECTS
The most commonly reported side effect is a generalized skin rash. Some children taking Cleocin may also experience diarrhea, nausea, vomiting, abdominal pain, jaundice, and, in rare cases, a severe allergic reaction (anaphylactic shock).

The manufacturer warns that the use of Cleocin has been associated with severe inflammation of the large intestine (colitis), which, in a few cases, has been fatal.

Codeine (generic)

BRAND NAMES
Codeine is a narcotic derived from opium and an ingredient in many prescription drugs, although when it is prescribed alone it is not marketed under a brand name.

PRODUCT CATEGORY
Analgesic/antitussive (cough suppressant).

DOSAGE FORM
Liquid and tablets.

WHY PRESCRIBED
This narcotic drug is used to relieve mild to moderate pain from a wide variety of causes. Under appropriate circumstances, it is also prescribed to help suppress troublesome coughing. Codeine is sometimes used in the short-term treatment of the symptoms of mild diarrhea.

CHILDREN'S DOSAGE
This depends largely on the condition being treated and the age and weight of the child. For example, the usual dosage for pain relief is 0.5 milligrams (1/10th of a teaspoonful) per kilogram of body weight (1 kilogram = 2.2 pounds), given four to six times daily. The usual dosage for cough suppression in children between the ages of six and twelve is 5 to 10 milligrams, given every four to six hours (up to a maximum total daily dosage of 60 mg).

PRECAUTIONS AND WARNINGS
Codeine can be habit-forming if it is taken for prolonged periods.

POSSIBLE SIDE EFFECTS
The most common side effects include constipation, drowsiness, nausea, vomiting, and dizziness. Large doses of codeine may cause potentially more serious side effects, such as respiratory depression.

Colace® (OTC)

GENERIC NAME
Docusate sodium.

PRODUCT CATEGORY
Stool softener.

DOSAGE FORM
Liquid (drops), syrup, and capsules.

WHY USED
It is used to soften stools in children who are constipated, thus helping reduce straining during bowel movement.

CHILDREN'S DOSAGE
Colace is available without a doctor's prescription. Administer to children exactly as the label recommends.

PRECAUTIONS AND WARNINGS
Although this product is available without a doctor's prescription, it is recommended that a physician be consulted about its use in the event the child has a health condition, such as a heart disease, that may be aggravated by straining during bowel movements. Colace is not a laxative and should not be used when constipation is due to a failure of peristalsis (normal intestinal contractions that move feces through the bowel).

Constipation in infants and small children is often related to dietary habits, such as ingesting large amounts of milk.

POSSIBLE SIDE EFFECTS
Side effects are relatively uncommon, but the child may experience a bitter taste, nausea, and throat irritation, particularly when the liquid or syrup forms of the product are used. Some cases of skin rash have been reported.

Combid®

GENERIC NAME
This product contains a combination of prochlorperazine maleate (10 mg) and isopropamide iodide (equivalent to 5 mg of isopropamide).

PRODUCT CATEGORY
Antispasmodic/antisecretory/antinauseant.

DOSAGE FORM
Capsules.

WHY PRESCRIBED
It is used to prevent or relieve muscular spasms of the stomach and intestines associated with various diseases and disorders of the gastrointestinal tract. Combid also reduces secretions from the stomach and helps control nausea and vomiting.

CHILDREN'S DOSAGE
Combid should not be given to children under the age of twelve years. For older children (and adults), the usual dosage is one capsule every twelve hours. Some children may require only one capsule daily to control symptoms.

PRECAUTIONS AND WARNINGS
Combid should be used with caution in children with jaundice, liver disease, or various disorders of the blood. Use of the drug may increase the sensitivity of a child to fever and heat stroke in a hot environment. Large doses may suppress intestinal activity in individuals with certain intestinal disorders.

POSSIBLE SIDE EFFECTS
The most commonly reported side effects include dry mouth, blurred vision, difficulty urinating, constipation, stuffy nose (nasal congestion), increase in heart rate (tachycardia), sensation of heartbeat (palpitations), dilation of pupils (mydriasis), drug-induced fever, and a bloated feeling.

Rarely, more serious side effects may be experienced. These include impairment of the blood-forming tissues, convulsions, and a severe drop in blood pressure.

Comhist®

GENERIC NAME
This product contains chlorpheniramine maleate (2 mg), phenylephrine hydrochloride (10 mg), and phenyltoloxamine citrate (25 mg).

PRODUCT CATEGORY
Antihistamine/decongestant.

DOSAGE FORM
Tablets.

WHY PRESCRIBED
Comhist is used to relieve the symptoms of runny nose and nasal congestion, particularly when associated with seasonal allergies such as hay fever. It works by shrinking swollen mucous membranes and increasing the air flow through the nasal passages.

CHILDREN'S DOSAGE
This product is not recommended for use in children under the age of six years. For children six to twelve years of age, the recommended dosage is one tablet every eight hours. For children twelve years and older, the recommended dosage is one or two tablets every eight hours.

PRECAUTIONS AND WARNINGS
Comhist should not be given to any child who is hypersensitive (allergic) to any of the ingredients in the product, or to children with heart disease, diabetes, high blood pressure, asthma, or certain other disorders, including abnormalities of the urinary and gastrointestinal tracts, without the advice and supervision of a physician. The product may interact with some other medications such as sedatives, hypnotics, and tranquilizers.

POSSIBLE SIDE EFFECTS
The most commonly reported side effects are urticaria (hives); skin rash; dryness of the mouth, nose, and throat; urinary retention or increased urge to urinate; nausea and vomiting; headache; sensation of heartbeat (palpitations); blurred vision; sedation; dizziness; nervousness and inability to fall asleep (insomnia).

Congespirin® Aspirin-Free Cold Tablets (OTC)

GENERIC NAME
This product contains a combination of acetaminophen (81 mg) and phenylephrine hydrochloride (1.25 mg).

PRODUCT CATEGORY
Analgesic (pain reliever)/decongestant.

DOSAGE FORM
Chewable tablets.

WHY USED
It is used to relieve symptoms of the common cold and flu, including fever, stuffy nose (nasal congestion), and minor aches and pains.

CHILDREN'S DOSAGE
This product is not recommended for use in children under the age of two years without the advice of a doctor. For older children, the following dosage is recommended:

Age of Child	Tablets Every Four Hours
2–3 years	2
4–5 years	3
6–8 years	4
9–10 years	5
11 years	6
12 years	8

Not more than four doses a day should be given without the advice of a physician.

PRECAUTIONS AND WARNINGS
Do not give Congespirin to children for more than ten days without the knowledge and advice of a physician. This drug should not be given to children with heart disease, thyroid disease, diabetes, high blood pressure (hypertension), or high fever, unless you are advised to do so by a physician.

POSSIBLE SIDE EFFECTS
Side effects are relatively uncommon. The phenylephrine hydrochloride ingredient may cause dryness or a burning sensation of the mucous membranes of the nose, headache, dizziness, nervousness, sensation of heartbeat (palpitations), and rapid heartbeat (tachycardia). It also may interact with caffeine beverages, such as colas, to increase the stimulation effect on the nervous system.

Congespirin® for Children Cough Syrup (OTC)

GENERIC NAME
This product contains dextromethorphan hydrobromide (5 mg per 5 ml teaspoonful).

PRODUCT CATEGORY
Antitussive.

DOSAGE FORM
Syrup (orange flavor).

WHY USED
This product is used to relieve the symptoms of coughs due to colds and minor throat irritations.

CHILDREN'S DOSAGE
Congespirin Cough Syrup should not be given to a child under the age of two years without the advice of a physician. For children between two and five years, the recommended dosage is one teaspoonful every four hours as needed. For children six to twelve years of age, the recommended dosage is two teaspoonfuls every four hours as needed. A child should not be given more than six doses in any 24-hour period.

PRECAUTIONS AND WARNINGS
Congespirin Cough Syrup should not be given to a child with a fever that continues for more than three days or a cough that persists for more than ten days without the advice of a physician. A persistent cough may be a symptom of a serious illness. The product also should not be given to a child under medical care without consulting a doctor. It should not be given to any child who has a known allergy to dextromethorphan.

POSSIBLE SIDE EFFECTS
Side effects are relatively uncommon but may include skin rash, drowsiness, nausea, diarrhea, or stomach pain.

Congespirin® for Children Liquid Cough Medicine (OTC)

GENERIC NAME
This product contains acetaminophen (130 mg), phenylpropanolamine hydrochloride (6.25 mg), and alcohol (10 percent) per 5 ml teaspoonful.

PRODUCT CATEGORY
Analgesic (pain reliever)/antipyretic (fever reducer)/decongestant.

DOSAGE FORM
Liquid.

WHY USED
This product is used to relieve the symptoms of fever, nasal congestion, and minor aches and pains associated with the common cold and flu.

CHILDREN'S DOSAGE
It is not recommended for use in children under the age of three years without the advice of a physician. For older children, the recommended dosage is:

Age of Child	Teaspoonfuls Every 3 or 4 Hours
3–5 years	1
6–12 years	2

The child should not be given more than four doses in any 24-hour period without the advice of a physician.

PRECAUTIONS AND WARNINGS
This product should not be given to any child under medical care without the physician's advice. It also should not be given to any child with heart disease, high blood pressure (hypertension), diabetes, thyroid disease, or a high fever, without a doctor's authorization. It also should not be continued for more than ten days without the advice of a physician.

POSSIBLE SIDE EFFECTS
This product is relatively free of side effects but it should not be given to a child with a known hypersensitivity (allergic reaction) to any of the ingredients. Side effects reported from the use of products containing phenylpropanolamine include headache, nervousness, paleness, rapid heartbeat (tachycardia), and difficulty in falling asleep (insomnia). The risk of side effects may be increased by using large doses of the drug.

Constant-T®

GENERIC NAME
Theophylline.

PRODUCT CATEGORY
Bronchodilator.

DOSAGE FORM
Tablets.

WHY PRESCRIBED
It is used to relieve and prevent symptoms of asthma and bronchospasm associated with chronic bronchitis.

CHILDREN'S DOSAGE
Because of a wide range of responses among various children of the same age and weight, the exact dosage needed to produce maximum relief of symptoms with a minimum risk of side effects should be determined by the child's physician.

PRECAUTIONS AND WARNINGS
Constant-T tablets should not be given to a child who is known to be hypersensitive (allergic) to theophylline or related substances. Blood levels of the drug should be monitored to ensure that doses are not excessive. Individual reactions can be influenced by a number of factors including liver and kidney function, heart disease, and fever. The drug may irritate the digestive tract of some children. Large doses may increase the risk of adverse effects.

POSSIBLE SIDE EFFECTS
The most commonly reported side effects include nausea, vomiting, diarrhea, headache, restlessness, sensation of heartbeat (palpitations), rapid heartbeat (tachycardia) and other abnormal heart rhythms, and rapid breathing. Because theophylline may interact with certain other medications, a doctor should be consulted if the child is taking other drugs.

Contac Jr.® (OTC)

GENERIC NAME
This product contains a combination of phenylpropanolamine hydrochloride (9.4 mg), acetaminophen (162.5 mg), dextromethorphan hydrobromide (5 mg), and alcohol (10 percent) in each 5 ml teaspoonful.

PRODUCT CATEGORY
Decongestant/analgesic (pain reliever)/antipyretic (fever reducer)/antitussive (cough suppressant).

DOSAGE FORM
Liquid.

WHY USED
Contac Jr. is used to relieve congestion, coughing, body aches, and fever associated with the common cold and flu.

CHILDREN'S DOSAGE
This product should not be given to a child who weighs less than 31 pounds or is less than three years old without the advice of a doctor. Individual dosage is based on the weight of the child as suggested on the label. Doses are given once every four hours with a maximum of six doses in any 24-hour period.

PRECAUTIONS AND WARNINGS
The dose given the child should not be larger than recommended on the label. If the symptoms persist for more than seven days or are accompanied by a high fever or severe or recurring pain, consult a doctor. The product should not be given to a child with heart disease or diabetes without the advice of a physician. Consult a doctor if the child is taking any other medication with the same ingredients.

POSSIBLE SIDE EFFECTS
Among the most commonly reported side effects are headache, nervousness, pale skin, difficulty in falling asleep (insomnia), and rapid heartbeat (tachycardia). Less frequent side effects are dizziness, difficulty urinating, loss of appetite, nausea, and vomiting.

Cordran®

GENERIC NAME
Flurandrenolide.

PRODUCT CATEGORY
Anti-inflammatory (corticosteroid).

DOSAGE FORM
Topical (for direct application to skin) cream, ointment, lotion, and adhesive tape.

WHY PRESCRIBED
It is used to treat various inflammatory disorders of the skin that respond to corticosteroid medications.

CHILDREN'S DOSAGE
The physician will give specific instructions for use of the product. In general, the ointment form of Cordran is used to treat dry or scaly areas of inflamed skin. Apply to the skin in a thin film two or three times daily. If the inflamed area is moist, the cream or lotion forms of the drug should be used. Rub gently into the affected skin two or three times daily.

PRECAUTIONS AND WARNINGS
Do not apply Cordran to areas of the child's skin that are infected. Not only does the drug have no beneficial effect on bacterial or fungal infections, but it may cause the disease to spread to nearby healthy areas of skin.

If Cordran causes a local irritation of the skin or if the inflammation seems to worsen, discontinue use of the drug and consult the physician.

This product should not be used on the skin of a child who has a known hypersensitivity (allergy) to corticosteroid drugs. Because potent corticosteroids can be absorbed through the skin and may affect certain hormones, prolonged or excessive use of such drugs may interfere with the normal growth and development of a child.

POSSIBLE SIDE EFFECTS
The most commonly reported side effects include itching, dry skin, skin eruptions, and a burning sensation at the site of drug application.

More serious side effects may occur if Cordran is applied to extensive areas of the skin or is left on for prolonged periods. However, this is less likely to occur if the child is under close medical supervision and the physician's instructions are closely followed.

Coricidin® Demilets® for Children (OTC)

GENERIC NAME
This product contains a combination of chlorpheniramine maleate (1 mg), acetaminophen (80 mg), and phenylpropanolamine hydrochloride (6.25 mg).

PRODUCT CATEGORY
Antihistamine/analgesic (pain reliever).

DOSAGE FORM
Tablets.

WHY USED
It is used for the relief of symptoms of the common cold, flu, and sinus trouble, including runny nose, stuffy nose, sneezing, watery eyes, itching eyes, fever, and minor aches and pains.

CHILDREN'S DOSAGE
This product should not be given to children under the age of six years without the advice of a physician. For children between six and eleven years, the recommended dosage is two tablets every four hours. The child should be given an adequate amount of water with each dose. The dosage should not exceed a total of twelve tablets in any 24-hour period without the advice of a physician.

PRECAUTIONS AND WARNINGS
This product should not be given to any child who is already taking another medication for high blood pressure, depression, appetite control, or other disorders without the advice of a physician. It also should not be given to a child with asthma, diabetes, heart disease, high blood pressure, thyroid disease, glaucoma, or difficulty urinating, except under the advice and supervision of a physician. Do not give the drug for more than five days. If fever is present or persists or recurs, limit use of the product to only three days. If the symptoms continue, or new ones develop, consult a physician.

POSSIBLE SIDE EFFECTS
The most commonly reported side effects include drowsiness, excitability, nervousness, sleeplessness, dizziness, or hypertension (high blood pressure). Large doses may result in severe liver damage.

Coricidin® Medilets® for Children (OTC)

GENERIC NAME
This product contains chlorpheniramine maleate (1 mg) and phenylpropanolamine hydrochloride (6.25 mg).

PRODUCT CATEGORY
Antihistamine/decongestant.

DOSAGE FORM
Tablets.

WHY USED
It is used for the relief of cold and sinus symptoms, including runny nose, sneezing, watery eyes, and itching eyes.

CHILDREN'S DOSAGE
Coricidin Medilets should not be given to children under the age of six years without the advice of a physician. For children between the ages of six and eleven, the recommended dosage is two tablets every four hours with a maximum total dosage of twelve tablets in a 24-hour period.

PRECAUTIONS AND WARNINGS
Use of this product should not be continued for more than seven days without the approval of a physician if symptoms do not improve or if they are accompanied by a high fever. The drug should not be given to children with asthma, glaucoma, high blood pressure, diabetes, heart disease, thyroid disease, or difficulty urinating. It should not be given to a child who is already receiving a medication for a more serious disorder, such as high blood pressure, depression, or appetite control, without the advice and supervision of a physician.

POSSIBLE SIDE EFFECTS
The most commonly reported side effects are drowsiness and excitability.

Cortisporin® Ophthalmic

GENERIC NAME
This product contains a combination of polymyxin B sulfate, bacitracin zinc (in ointment only), neomycin sulfate, and hydrocortisone.

PRODUCT CATEGORY
Ophthalmic (eye) preparation/antibiotic/corticosteroid.

DOSAGE FORM
Ointment and suspension.

WHY PRESCRIBED
It is used to treat infections of the eye caused by bacteria that are susceptible to the drug's ingredients.

CHILDREN'S DOSAGE
This depends on the severity of the infection. Usually, the ointment is applied every three or four hours. The physician will give detailed instructions on the use of either form of this product.

PRECAUTIONS AND WARNINGS
Stop giving this product and consult the doctor if there is an increase in local irritation of the eye or eyelid or evidence of an allergic reaction. (Some children may be especially allergic to the neomycin ingredient.) Should this occur, consult the physician immediately.

POSSIBLE SIDE EFFECTS
Prolonged use of any antibiotic can cause the growth and multiplication of microorganisms that are unaffected by the drug. Such a "superinfection" may occur with the long-term use of Cortisporin Ophthalmic.

The most common side effect in short-term therapy with this drug is an allergic reaction in children who are especially sensitive to neomycin.

Cortisporin® Otic

GENERIC NAME
This product contains a combination of polymyxin B sulfate, neomycin sulfate, and hydrocortisone.

PRODUCT CATEGORY
Otic (ear) preparation/antibiotic/corticosteroid.

DOSAGE FORM
Liquid solution or suspension (instilled with a dropper directly into the outer ear canal).

WHY PRESCRIBED
It is used to treat susceptible bacterial infections that involve the outer ear canal.

CHILDREN'S DOSAGE
The physician will give detailed instructions on the use of this product. The usual dosage for infants and children is three drops instilled into the affected ear three or four times daily. The child should remain with the affected ear upward for five minutes to permit the drops to spread throughout the ear canal. Caution should be used if the medication is warmed before application to make sure it is not warmer than body temperature as excessive heat can reduce the potency of the drug.

PRECAUTIONS AND WARNINGS
Some children may experience an allergic skin reaction, characterized by redness and swelling. Itching and dry scaling of the skin may also be a problem.

If the child complains of a sharp stinging or burning sensation, consult the doctor at once. This may be caused by a perforated eardrum, which requires medical attention.

Children's CoTYLENOL® Liquid Cold Formula (OTC)

GENERIC NAME
This product contains in each 5 ml teaspoonful acetaminophen (160 mg), chlorpheniramine maleate (1 mg), phenylpropanolamine hydrochloride (6.25 mg), and alcohol (8.5 percent).

PRODUCT CATEGORY
Analgesic (pain reliever)/antipyretic (fever reducer)/antihistamine/decongestant.

DOSAGE FORM
Liquid (cherry flavored).

WHY USED
It is used to relieve the symptoms of the common cold and flu. These include stuffy nose (nasal congestion), runny nose, sneezing, fever, and general muscular aches and pains.

CHILDREN'S DOSAGE
Children's CoTYLENOL Liquid Cold Formula should not be given to children under the age of six years unless directed by a physician. The usual dosage for children between the ages of two and five years is one teaspoonful (5 ml) every four to six hours as needed. Children between six and eleven may receive two teaspoonfuls (10 ml) every four to six hours. Children twelve years and older usually receive four teaspoonfuls (20 ml) every six hours. Do not exceed four doses within a period of 24 hours.

PRECAUTIONS AND WARNINGS
Do not give this product to children with high blood pressure (hypertension), diabetes, heart disorders, or thyroid disease without the advice of a physician.

POSSIBLE SIDE EFFECTS
The most commonly reported side effects include drowsiness, nervousness, restlessness, or the inability to fall asleep (insomnia). Overdosage with this product can cause serious damage to the liver.

Children's CoTYLENOL®
Chewable Cold Tablets (OTC)

GENERIC NAME
This product contains in each tablet acetaminophen (80 mg), chlorpheniramine maleate (0.5 mg), and phenylpropanolamine hydrochloride (3.125 mg).

PRODUCT CATEGORY
Analgesic (pain reliever)/antipyretic (fever reducer)/antihistamine/decongestant.

DOSAGE FORM
Chewable tablets.

WHY USED
It is used to relieve the symptoms of the common cold or flu: stuffy nose (nasal congestion), runny nose, sneezing, fever, and general muscular aches and pains.

CHILDREN'S DOSAGE
Children's CoTYLENOL Chewable Tablets should not be given to children under the age of six years unless directed by a physician. The usual dosage for children between the ages of two and five years is two tablets every four to six hours as needed. Children between six and eleven years may be given four tablets every four to six hours. Children of any age should not receive more than four doses in any 24-hour period.

PRECAUTIONS AND WARNINGS
Do not give this product to children with high blood pressure (hypertension), diabetes, heart disorders, or thyroid disease without the advice of a physician. CoTYLENOL Chewable Cold Tablets contain aspartame, which may produce an adverse reaction in a child with phenylketonuria (PKU).

POSSIBLE SIDE EFFECTS
The most commonly reported side effects include drowsiness, nervousness, restlessness, or the inability to fall asleep (insomnia). Overdosage with this product can cause serious damage to the liver.

Cremacoat® 3 (OTC)

GENERIC NAME
This product contains a combination of dextromethorphan hydrobromide (20 mg), phenylpropanolamine hydrochloride (37.5 mg), and guaifenesin (200 mg) per three teaspoonful (15 ml) dose, and alcohol (10 percent).

PRODUCT CATEGORY
Antitussive (relieves coughing)/decongestant/expectorant.

DOSAGE FORM
Liquid (raspberry flavor).

WHY USED
It is used to relieve the symptoms of coughing, nasal congestion, and throat irritation associated with the common cold and to loosen phlegm and mucus in the upper respiratory passages of the throat and chest.

CHILDREN'S DOSAGE
Cremacoat 3 is available without a doctor's prescription. Administer to children exactly as the label recommends. Note that this drug should not be given to children under the age of two years without the advice of a physician.

PRECAUTIONS AND WARNINGS
This product should not be given to children with diabetes, heart disease, high blood pressure, or to a child with a high fever or persistent cough unless advised by a doctor.

POSSIBLE SIDE EFFECTS
Side effects from the use of this product are infrequent, but use of large doses may result in restlessness, anxiety, sweating, tremor, rapid heartbeat (tachycardia) and other heartbeat abnormalities, high blood pressure, confusion, nausea, and vomiting.

Cylert®

GENERIC NAME
Pemoline.

PRODUCT CATEGORY
Central nervous system stimulant.

DOSAGE FORM
Tablets (18.75 mg, 37.5 mg, and 75 mg). It is also available in 37.5 mg chewable tablets.

WHY PRESCRIBED
It is used in the treatment of children diagnosed as having attention deficit disorder (ADD)—previously known as minimal brain dysfunction (MBD)—with hyperactivity. The condition may be characterized by emotional instability, impulsiveness, severe distractibility, and short attention span.

CHILDREN'S DOSAGE
Cylert is given as a single dose each morning. The usual starting dose is 37.5 milligrams per day, with gradual increases of 18.75 milligrams at intervals of one week until a daily maximum dosage of 112.5 milligrams (three 37.5 milligram tablets) is reached or until the desired response is achieved.

PRECAUTIONS AND WARNINGS
Cylert should never be given to children under the age of six. It should not be given to children with impaired kidney or liver function without the advice of a doctor.

POSSIBLE SIDE EFFECTS
The most commonly reported side effect is insomnia. In some children, the drug may aggravate symptoms of behavior disturbance and thought disorders, or it may cause convulsive seizures, hallucinations, mild depression, increased irritability, dizziness, drowsiness, or other changes involving the nervous system. Skin rash, digestive upsets with loss of appetite and weight loss, and retarded growth rate also have been reported.

Dalmane®

GENERIC NAME
Flurazepam hydrochloride.

PRODUCT CATEGORY
Hypnotic agent (sleep-inducing drug).

DOSAGE FORM
Capsules.

WHY PRESCRIBED
It is used to help induce restful sleep in those who have difficulty in falling asleep and those who wake up frequently during the night.

CHILDREN'S DOSAGE
Dalmane is not recommended for use in children under the age of fifteen years. The dosage for older children (and adults) will be determined by the physician based on the needs of the individual patient.

PRECAUTIONS AND WARNINGS
Prolonged use of Dalmane can lead to psychological dependence on the drug. Potentially dangerous sedative effects may occur if Dalmane is taken together with alcohol or other drugs having a tranquilizing effect. Such drug interactions can have an additive effect that may continue for several days, as can excessive doses of Dalmane, leading to confusion and coma. Thus, the patient should avoid such combinations and should use caution when engaging in tasks that require mental alertness.

POSSIBLE SIDE EFFECTS
The most common side effects include dizziness, drowsiness, impaired coordination, lightheadedness, headache, heartburn, nausea, vomiting, diarrhea, severe sedation, and disorientation.

Datril® Extra Strength (OTC)

GENERIC NAME
Acetaminophen.

PRODUCT CATEGORY
Analgesic (pain reliever)/antipyretic (fever reducer).

DOSAGE FORM
Tablets and capsules (500 mg).

WHY USED
It is used to relieve symptoms of fever, headaches, and other minor aches and pains.

CHILDREN'S DOSAGE
This product is not recommended for children under the age of 12 years. The usual recommended dosage for older children (and adults) is two tablets or capsules every four hours if needed. Do not exceed the recommended daily maximum of eight tablets or capsules.

PRECAUTIONS AND WARNINGS
This drug should not be given to any child who has shown a hypersensitivity (allergy) to acetaminophen products. If an allergic reaction occurs, discontinue use of the drug and consult a doctor. Datril should not be given to a child under medical care without the advice of a physician. A physician also should be consulted if the child has severe or continued pain or a high or continued fever.

POSSIBLE SIDE EFFECTS
There have been few reports of side effects from the use of acetaminophen, but a child may experience a skin rash or a sore tongue (glossitis) after use of the product.

Deltasone®

GENERIC NAME
Prednisone.

PRODUCT CATEGORY
Corticosteroid (synthetic glucocorticoid)/anti-inflammatory.

DOSAGE FORM
Tablets.

WHY PRESCRIBED
It is used in the treatment of a wide variety of inflammatory diseases of the skin; rheumatic disorders (such as juvenile rheumatoid arthritis, psoriatic arthritis, and ankylosing spondylitis); collagen diseases (including systemic lupus erythematosus); allergies (including bronchial asthma and contact dermatitis); lung diseases; specific blood disorders; and several other conditions.

Deltasone is often used in combination with other corticosteroids in treating disorders of the adrenal glands (such as Addison's disease) to replace hormones normally produced by these glands.

CHILDREN'S DOSAGE
This depends on the type and severity of the condition being treated and the response of the child to Deltasone. The physician will adjust the dosage to each child's requirements.

PRECAUTIONS AND WARNINGS
Children should not be vaccinated against smallpox or be subjected to other immunization procedures while undergoing corticosteroid therapy. Because Deltasone may interact with aspirin and many other prescription and nonprescription drugs, resulting in adverse effects, the doctor should be consulted about giving the child any additional medications while taking this product. Prednisone products may affect a child's response to surgery, injury, or illness for up to two years after the drug has been discontinued. Thus, any doctor providing care for the child in the next two years should be advised of the child's previous use of the drug.

POSSIBLE SIDE EFFECTS
All drugs in the general class of corticosteroids, such as Deltasone, are capable of a wide range of side effects. These are largely related to the dosage and the duration of therapy. Among the reported side effects are suppressed growth in children; accumulation of fatty deposits around the face, neck, or abdomen; nervousness; thinning of the bone structure (osteoporosis); increased susceptibility to infection; water retention, resulting in a swelling of the tissues (edema); euphoria; difficulty in falling asleep (insomnia); skin changes; and increased susceptibility to bruising.

Demerol®

GENERIC NAME
Meperidine hydrochloride.

PRODUCT CATEGORY
Narcotic analgesic.

DOSAGE FORM
Syrup (banana flavor), and tablets.

WHY PRESCRIBED
It is used mainly to provide quick relief from moderate to severe pain due to a wide variety of causes.

CHILDREN'S DOSAGE
This depends on the severity of the pain, the body weight of the child, and the child's response to Demerol. The usual dosage is 1 to 1.8 milligrams per kilogram of body weight (1 kilogram = 2.2 pounds) given every three or four hours, as required.

PRECAUTIONS AND WARNINGS
Demerol is a narcotic analgesic and has the ability to cause addiction or drug dependence if it is taken for prolonged periods. Excessive doses may also cause convulsions.

POSSIBLE SIDE EFFECTS
The most commonly reported side effects include dizziness, lightheadedness, sedation, nausea, vomiting, and sweating. More serious side effects such as slow and ineffective breathing (respiratory depression), sudden drop in blood pressure, and stopping of the heart (cardiac arrest) and occasionally seen in some patients.

Desitin® Ointment (OTC)

GENERIC NAME
This product contains a combination of zinc oxide (40 percent), cod liver oil, and talc in a petrolatum-lanolin base.

PRODUCT CATEGORY
Emollient (softener)/antiburn medication.

DOSAGE FORM
Ointment.

WHY USED
It is used to relieve symptoms of chafed skin, diaper rash, and other superficial skin injuries, including minor cuts, abrasions, burns, and irritations, by forming a temporary protective barrier over the affected area.

CHILDREN'S DOSAGE
Desitin Ointment is available without a doctor's prescription. Administer to the child according to the instructions on the label, which vary with the specific use.

PRECAUTIONS AND WARNINGS
Desitin is intended for external use only. Do not use this product on a child who has a known hypersensitivity (allergy) to any of the ingredients. If a reaction occurs, discontinue use of the product and consult a physician. Consult a physician if any of the symptoms continue or worsen.

POSSIBLE SIDE EFFECTS
No serious side effects have been reported from use of Desitin Ointment.

Dexedrine®

GENERIC NAME
Dextroamphetamine sulfate.

PRODUCT CATEGORY
Central nervous system stimulant.

DOSAGE FORM
Capsules (sustained-release), tablets, and elixir.

WHY PRESCRIBED
It is used mainly in the treatment of attention deficit disorder (ADD)—formerly known as minimal brain dysfunction (MBD)—with hyperactivity in children. The condition is marked by a short attention span, easy distractibility, impulsiveness, and emotional instability. The product is also used in the treatment of narcolepsy (an inability to remain awake) and in certain serious cases of obesity.

CHILDREN'S DOSAGE
Amphetamines are not recommended for use in children under the age of three years for attention deficit disorder with hyperactivity, or as an appetite suppressant in children under the age of twelve years. For children between the ages of three and five years, the usual recommended dosage for attention deficit disorder with hyperactivity is 2.5 milligrams daily in tablets or elixir at first, with gradual increases of 2.5 milligrams daily at weekly intervals, until a physician determines that a proper response has been reached. For children six years and older, the initial daily dosage may be 5 milligrams once or twice a day, with increases of 5 milligrams a day at weekly intervals, until a physician determines that a proper response has been reached. With rare exceptions, the total daily dose should not exceed 40 milligrams. The first dose is given on awakening, and any additional doses are given after intervals of four to six hours. The doctor may recommend occasional interruptions of therapy to see whether any symptoms of attention deficit disorder recur when the drug is not used.

PRECAUTIONS AND WARNINGS
Because amphetamines are potentially habit-forming, they should be used for appetite control only when other measures have failed. The drug should not be given to a child with heart disease, high blood pressure, or thyroid disease, nor to a child who is known to be hypersensitive to this product or similar drugs without the advice and supervision of a physician. In general, the dosage used should be the least amount needed to produce the desired medical benefits in order to reduce the risk of overdosage. In children with serious mental disorders, amphetamines may aggravate thought disorders and behavior disturbances.

POSSIBLE SIDE EFFECTS
Among the reported side effects in children are tics and other automatic (involuntary) activity of nerves and muscles. Other side effects may include increased blood pressure, sensation of heartbeat (palpitations), rapid heartbeat (tachycardia), restlessness, dizziness, tremors, difficulty in falling asleep (insomnia), headaches, urticaria (hives), dryness of the mouth, loss of appetite and weight loss, and digestive system disorders such as constipation and diarrhea.

Dilantin®

GENERIC NAME
Phenytoin.

PRODUCT CATEGORY
Anticonvulsant (antiepileptic).

DOSAGE FORM
Pediatric suspension, chewable tablets (Infatabs), and capsules (as the sodium salt).

WHY PRESCRIBED
It is mainly used to prevent grand mal epileptic seizures or to reduce the frequency of convulsive attacks.

CHILDREN'S DOSAGE
The usual initial daily dosage for children is 5 milligrams per kilogram of body weight (1 kilogram = 2.2 pounds), given on the first day of treatment in two or three equally divided doses. Thereafter, the recommended total daily dosages may range between 4 and 8 milligrams per kilogram of body weight, adjusted by the physician according to the needs and response of the individual child. The doctor also may recommend the minimum adult daily dose of 300 milligrams for children over six years of age.

PRECAUTIONS AND WARNING
This product should not be given to a child who is hypersensitive (allergic) to phenytoin or similar drugs. If a skin rash develops, the prescribing physician should be notified immediately. Do not suddenly discontinue use of Dilantin. If the drug must be discontinued altogether because of an adverse reaction, the physician will substitute another antiepileptic drug as rapidly as is feasible. Sudden withdrawal of the drug may trigger a serious convulsive condition known as status epilepticus.

Do not give the child aspirin or any other drugs during therapy with Dilantin without the advice of a physician.

POSSIBLE SIDE EFFECTS
The most commonly reported side effects include impaired muscular coordination (ataxia), involuntary movement of the eyeballs (nystagmus), slurred speech, mental confusion, dizziness, headache, skin rash, nausea, vomiting, constipation, and swelling of the gums. Many symptoms involving the central nervous system may be due to excessive doses of the drug. More serious side effects, such as impairment of the blood-forming tissues, occur much less frequently. Phenytoin may alter blood sugar levels in diabetic patients, and it can interfere with vitamin D metabolism, affecting normal bone development.

Dimetane®, Dimetane® Decongestant (OTC)

GENERIC NAME
This product contains a combination of brompheniramine maleate, phenylephrine hydrochloride (in Decongestant), and alcohol (in elixir form).

PRODUCT CATEGORY
Antihistamine/decongestant.

DOSAGE FORM
Tablets and elixir.

WHY USED
It is used to relieve the symptoms of runny nose, sneezing, itching of the nose, throat, and eyes, nasal congestion, and watery eyes associated with the common cold and allergies such as hay fever.

CHILDREN'S DOSAGE
This product is not recommended for use in children under the age of two years. For children between the ages of six and twelve years, the usual recommended dosage is ½ tablet every four hours, with a maximum total daily dosage of three tablets; for children twelve years of age and older, the recommended dosage is one tablet every four hours, with a maximum total daily dosage of six tablets.

The recommended dosage for the elixir form is:

Age of Child	Teaspoonfuls (5 ml) Every 4 Hours
2–6 years	½
6–12 years	1
12 years and over	2

The daily total should not exceed six doses.

PRECAUTIONS AND WARNINGS
Do not give Dimetane to a child who is known to be hypersensitive (allergic) to any of the ingredients. The product may cause excitability in children. It should not be given to a child with asthma, glaucoma, high blood pressure, heart disease, diabetes, or thyroid disease. The doctor should be consulted if the child is taking any other medication that may interact with Dimetane.

POSSIBLE SIDE EFFECTS
The most commonly reported side effects include sedation, drowsiness, disturbed coordination, dizziness, nervousness, sleeplessness, or hives (urticaria). Side effects are most likely to result from giving larger than recommended dosages.

Dimetapp® (OTC)

GENERIC NAME
This product contains in each teaspoonful (5 ml) brompheniramine maleate (2 mg), phenylpropanolamine hydrochloride (12.5 mg), and alcohol (2.3 percent).

PRODUCT CATEGORY
Antihistamine/decongestant.

DOSAGE FORM
Elixir (grape flavor). Also available as tablets containing brompheniramine maleate (4 mg) and phenylpropanolamine hydrochloride (25 mg.)

WHY USED
It is used to relieve the symptoms of hay fever (allergic rhinitis), including stuffy nose (nasal congestion) and runny nose.

CHILDREN'S DOSAGE
The usual recommended dosage is:

Age of Child	Teaspoonfuls (5 ml) 3–4 Times Daily
1–6 months	¼
7 months–2 years	½
2–4 years	¾
4–12 years	1

PRECAUTIONS AND WARNINGS
Dimetapp Elixir should not be given to newborn or premature infants or used to treat children who have bronchial asthma or other disorders of the lower part of the respiratory tract. Do not give this drug to children who are hypersensitive (allergic) to antihistamines.

POSSIBLE SIDE EFFECTS
The most commonly reported side effects include sedation, drowsiness, sensation of the heartbeat (palpitations), disturbed coordination, dizziness, thickening of the secretions in the lower air passages, drug-induced skin rash, hives (urticaria), chills, dryness of the nose and throat, and wheezing.

More severe side effects are infrequent. In infants and children, an overdosage of antihistamines may cause hallucinations, convulsions, or even death.

Domeboro® (OTC)

GENERIC NAME
This product contains aluminum sulfate and calcium acetate.

PRODUCT CATEGORY
Astringent wet dressing

DOSAGE FORM
Tablet or powder (to be dissolved in water).

WHY USED
This product is used to relieve the symptoms of skin inflammation resulting from insect bites, poison ivy, athlete's foot, and minor bruises and swelling.

CHILDREN'S DOSAGE
This product is available without a doctor's prescription. It should be used according to the instructions supplied by the manufacturer.

PRECAUTIONS AND WARNINGS
This product is intended for external use only. Do not allow the dry or dissolved chemicals to come in contact with the eyes. Application of the dissolved medication to the wet bandages should be continued for four to eight hours, unless otherwise instructed by the physician. If any adverse reaction occurs, discontinue use of the product and contact a physician immediately.

POSSIBLE SIDE EFFECTS
No serious side effects have been reported from the use of this product.

Donnagel® (OTC)

GENERIC NAME
This product contains a combination of kaolin, pectin, hyoscyamine sulfate, atropine sulfate, scopolamine hydrobromide, and alcohol (3.8 percent).

PRODUCT CATEGORY
Antidiarrheal.

DOSAGE FORM
Liquid (oral suspension).

WHY USED
It is used to control common diarrhea.

CHILDREN'S DOSAGE
Do not give Donnagel to children under the age of three years unless advised to do so by a physician. This product is available without a doctor's prescription. Administer to children exactly as the label recommends.

PRECAUTIONS AND WARNINGS
If the child has severe or prolonged diarrhea, see a doctor at once so that a more serious underlying problem can be ruled out or diagnosed and treated. Do not give a child this product for more than two days in the presence of a high fever.

Do not give Donnagel to children with heart disorders, asthma, or other chronic illnesses without medical advice.

POSSIBLE SIDE EFFECTS
Used as directed, Donnagel is relatively free from adverse effects.

Donnatal®

GENERIC NAME
This product contains in each teaspoonful (5 ml), capsule, or tablet a combination of phenobarbital (16.2 mg), hyoscyamine sulfate (0.1037 mg), atropine sulfate (0.0194 mg), scopolamine hydrobromide (0.0065 mg), and alcohol (23 percent in elixir).

PRODUCT CATEGORY
Antispasmodic/mild sedative.

DOSAGE FORM
Elixir, capsules, and tablets.

WHY PRESCRIBED
It is used to relieve muscular spasms of the stomach and intestines associated with various disorders of the gastrointestinal tract. Donnatal also provides a mild sedative effect.

CHILDREN'S DOSAGE
This depends on the severity of the symptoms, the body weight of the child, the frequency of use and the child's response to Donnatal therapy. The physician will adjust the dosage according to the needs of the individual child to assure relief of symptoms with the least possibility of side effects.

PRECAUTIONS AND WARNINGS
Donnatal should not be given to children suffering from chronic lung disease.

The phenobarbital component of Donnatal can be habit-forming if it is taken in excessive amounts for prolonged periods. However, this is unlikely because of the relatively small amount of the drug in this product.

POSSIBLE SIDE EFFECTS
The most commonly reported side effects include dry mouth, difficulty urinating, dryness of the skin, flushing, and blurred vision. These side effects are ordinarily related to taking an excessive amount of the drug.

Dorcol® Children's Fever & Pain Reducer (OTC)

GENERIC NAME
This product contains in each teaspoonful (5 ml) acetaminophen (160 mg), alcohol (10 percent), edetate disodium, benzoic acid, and various other ingredients, including flavorings and colorings.

PRODUCT CATEGORY
Analgesic (pain reliever)/antipyretic (fever reducer).

DOSAGE FORM
Liquid.

WHY USED
This product is used to relieve symptoms of pain and fever in infants and children.

CHILDREN'S DOSAGE
This product is not recommended for use in children under the age of two years without the advice of a physician, who will determine a specific number of drops per kilogram of body weight (1 kilogram = 2.2 pounds) of the infant or child. For older children, the usual recommended dosage is by age or weight of the child, according to the following schedule:

Age of Child	Teaspoonfuls (5 ml) Every Four Hours
2–4 years	1
4–6 years	1½
6 years and over	2

Body Weight	Teaspoonfuls (5 ml) Every Four Hours
25–35 pounds	1
36–45 pounds	1½
46–60 pounds	2

Unless directed by a physician, the child should not be given more than five doses in any 24-hour period.

PRECAUTIONS AND WARNINGS
This product should not be given to a child with a known hypersensitivity to acetaminophen or the other ingredients. It should not be given to children with anemia or kidney or liver disease without the advice of a physician. Children are more sensitive than adults to an effect of acetaminophen on the red blood cells.

POSSIBLE SIDE EFFECTS
Acetaminophen, when used according to directions, is relatively free of side effects. However, some hypersensitivity reactions have been reported with occasional skin rashes and urticaria (hives).

Dorcol® Children's Liquid Cold Formula (OTC)

GENERIC NAME
This product contains in each teaspoonful (5 ml) pseudoephedrine hydrochloride (15 mg), chlorpheniramine maleate (1 mg), benzoic acid, and other ingredients, including flavorings and colorings.

PRODUCT CATEGORY
Decongestant/antihistamine.

DOSAGE FORM
Liquid.

WHY USED
It is used to relieve symptoms of nasal congestion, runny nose, and sinus pressure associated with the common cold, hay fever, and other common respiratory allergies.

CHILDREN'S DOSAGE
This product is not recommended for use in children under six years of age without the advice of a physician, who will prescribe a specific number of drops or teaspoonfuls according to the age and body weight of the infant or child. For children between six and twelve years of age weighing between 45 and 85 pounds, the usual recommended dosage is two teaspoonfuls every four to six hours, with a maximum of four doses in any 24-hour period.

PRECAUTIONS AND WARNINGS
This product should not be given to any child with a known hypersensitivity (allergy) to any of the ingredients. It also should not be used to treat symptoms of the lower respiratory tract. Antihistamines should not be given to premature or newborn infants. A doctor should be consulted before giving the drug to a child with high blood pressure, heart disease, diabetes, thyroid disease, or glaucoma.

POSSIBLE SIDE EFFECTS
Reported side effects include drowsiness, blurred vision, mild central nervous system stimulation, dry mouth, rapid heartbeat (tachycardia), dizziness, and digestive disorders. The product also may result in a thickening of secretions in the bronchial tubes (air passages leading to the lungs).

Dramamine® (OTC)

GENERIC NAME
Dimenhydrinate.

PRODUCT CATEGORY
Antiemetic/antihistamine.

DOSAGE FORM
Liquid and tablets.

WHY USED
It is used for the prevention or control of the symptoms of motion sickness, including nausea, vomiting, and vertigo.

CHILDREN'S DOSAGE
Dramamine is available without a doctor's prescription. It should be administered to children exactly as the label recommends. This product is not recommended for children under the age of two years without medical approval. For motion sickness, the drug should be given between thirty minutes and one hour before the start of travel or other activity that may produce symptoms.

PRECAUTIONS AND WARNINGS
Dramamine should not be used as the same time as antibiotics without first checking with the prescribing physician. Some antibiotics (such as streptomycin or kanamycin) can cause potentially severe damage to the inner parts of the ear (ototoxicity), the early symptoms of which may be masked by the use of Dramamine.

POSSIBLE SIDE EFFECTS
The most common side effect is relatively mild drowsiness.

Dristan® Advanced Formula (OTC)

GENERIC NAME
This product contains a combination of phenylephrine hydrochloride (5 mg), chlorpheniramine maleate (2 mg), acetaminophen (325 mg), and various other ingredients, including coloring.

PRODUCT CATEGORY
Decongestant/antihistamine/analgesic (pain reliever/antipyretic (fever reducer).

DOSAGE FORM
Tablets.

WHY USED
This product is used to relieve the symptoms of nasal congestion, sneezing, runny nose, fever, headache, and minor aches and pains associated with the common cold, flu, hay fever, or other allergies involving the upper respiratory tract.

CHILDREN'S DOSAGE
This product is not recommended for use in children under the age of six years. For children between the ages of six and twelve, the usual recommended dosage is one tablet every four hours. For children over twelve (and adults), the usual dosage is two tablets every four hours. No more than six doses should be taken in any 24-hour period.

PRECAUTIONS AND WARNINGS
This product may cause drowsiness or excitability in children. It should not be given to a child with asthma, glaucoma, high blood pressure, diabetes, heart disease, or thyroid disease without the advice of a physician. Do not continue using the drug more than seven days if symptoms do not subside or if the child has a high fever, unless advised to do so by a physician.

POSSIBLE SIDE EFFECTS
Reported side effects include nervousness, dizziness, and sleeplessness, particularly when larger than recommended doses are taken.

Drixoral® (OTC)

GENERIC NAME
This product contains a combination of dexbrompheniramine maleate and pseudoephedrine sulfate.

PRODUCT CATEGORY
Decongestant/antihistamine.

DOSAGE FORM
Sustained-action tablets, elixir.

WHY USED
It is mainly used to relieve the symptoms of stuffy nose (nasal congestion) associated with allergies such as hay fever (allergic rhinitis). Drixoral is also used to unblock a congested eustachian tube—the canal between the middle ear and the upper part of the throat that equalizes air pressure on either side of the eardrum.

CHILDREN'S DOSAGE
Drixoral tablets should not be given to children under the age of twelve years. For older children (and adults), the usual dosage is one tablet in the morning and one tablet at bedtime.

PRECAUTIONS AND WARNINGS
Drixoral should be used with caution (if at all) in children with high blood pressure, thyroid disease, heart disorders, or diabetes.

POSSIBLE SIDE EFFECTS
The most commonly reported side effects include drowsiness, restlessness, nausea, vomiting, skin rashes, dizziness, sensation of heartbeat (palpitations), headache, insomnia, difficulty urinating, rapid heartbeat (tachycardia), and abdominal cramps.

Dynapen®

GENERIC NAME
Dicloxacillin sodium.

PRODUCT CATEGORY
Antibiotic (semisynthetic penicillin).

DOSAGE FORM
Liquid (oral suspension) and capsules.

WHY PRESCRIBED
It is mainly used to treat specific types of bacterial infections (those caused by staphylococci that are resistant to penicillin).

CHILDREN'S DOSAGE
This depends largely on the severity of the infection, its site, and the weight of the child. For example, the usual dosage recommended to treat severe infections of the lower part of the respiratory tract—in children who weigh less than 40 kilograms (88 pounds)—is at least 25 milligrams per kilogram of body weight per day, in equally divided doses given every six hours. For a mild to moderate infection of the lower respiratory tract, the children's dosage may be only half that amount every six hours.

PRECAUTIONS AND WARNINGS
Dynapen should never be given to a child with a known allergic reaction to it or to penicillin. Adverse reactions are more likely if the child has experienced other allergies such as hay fever or hives (urticaria) or has asthma.

Long-term use of any antibiotic may result in the development of a "superinfection"—the growth and multiplication in the body of fungi and other microorganisms that are not affected by the drug.

Dispose of any remaining suspension or capsules of Dynapen once the course of therapy has been successfully completed.

POSSIBLE SIDE EFFECTS
Some children taking Dynapen may experience nausea, vomiting, diarrhea, or skin rashes. More serious side effects are relatively uncommon.

E.E.S.®

GENERIC NAME
Erythromycin ethylsuccinate.

PRODUCT CATEGORY
Antibiotic.

DOSAGE FORM
Oral suspension, tablets, chewable tablets (cherry flavor).

WHY PRESCRIBED
This product is used in the treatment of various infections of the skin, upper and lower respiratory tracts, and other body tissues, including those of the urinary tract and digestive system.

CHILDREN'S DOSAGE
This depends largely on the age and weight of the child and the severity of the infection. In general, the physician may prescribe 30 milligrams to 50 milligrams of the drug daily, to be given in divided doses, for each kilogram of body weight (1 kilogram = 2.2 pound) of the child. For severe infections, the amount of antibiotic to be given each day may be doubled by the physician.

PRECAUTIONS AND WARNINGS
Erythromycin should not be given to a child with a known hypersensitivity (allergy) to this drug. Caution is advised in giving the drug to a child with impaired liver function. If the child is taking another type of medication, the doctor should be advised because of the risk of an adverse reaction between incompatible drugs. Long-term use of any antibiotic may result in the development of a "superinfection"—the growth and multiplication in the body of fungi and other microorganisms that are not affected by the drug.

POSSIBLE SIDE EFFECTS
Among side effects reported from the use of erythromycin drugs in children are digestive upsets, with diarrhea, nausea, vomiting, and abdominal cramps; mild skin rashes and urticaria (hives); liver disorders with or without jaundice; and temporary hearing loss, which may be due to the use of large doses.

Elixophyllin®

GENERIC NAME
Theophylline.

PRODUCT CATEGORY
Bronchodilator.

DOSAGE FORM
Elixir and capsules.

WHY PRESCRIBED
Elixophyllin is used to relax the bronchial tubes and other tissues of the lungs, thereby relieving the symptoms of asthma, chronic bronchitis, and other breathing disorders.

CHILDREN'S DOSAGE
This product is not recommended for use in children less than six months old. The use of the capsule form of the drug is not recommended for children under the age of six years. The exact dosage depends upon various individual factors such as the age and weight of the child and the particular needs and response of the child to the therapy. The child should take only the prescribed dose and only at the time interval prescribed by the physician.

PRECAUTIONS AND WARNINGS
This product should not be given to a child who has a known hypersensitivity (allergy) to theophylline. It should not be taken along with any other medication containing theophylline or a substance chemically related to it. It should be given to a child with a heart disorder, liver disease, high blood pressure, or thyroid disease only with the advice and supervision of a physician. The drug may act as an irritant to the digestive tract in some individuals.

POSSIBLE SIDE EFFECTS
The most commonly reported side effects are nausea, vomiting, diarrhea, abdominal pain, headache, irritability, restlessness, excitability, difficulty in falling asleep (insomnia), convulsions, and heartbeat abnormalities, including rapid heartbeat (tachycardia), sensation of heartbeat (palpitations), and heart rhythm disorders (arrhythmias).

Emetrol® (OTC)

GENERIC NAME
This product is a combination of levulose (fructose), dextrose (glucose), and orthophosphoric acid.

PRODUCT CATEGORY
Antiemetic (phosphorated carbohydrate).

DOSAGE FORM
Liquid (mint flavor).

WHY USED
It is mainly used to relieve the symptoms of nausea and vomiting associated with motion sickness, "stomach flu," drug therapy, and other conditions, including regurgitation by infants.

CHILDREN'S DOSAGE
Emetrol is available without a doctor's prescription. Administer to children exactly as the label recommends. Do not give the child any other liquids for at least fifteen minutes before or after giving Emetrol.

PRECAUTIONS AND WARNINGS
If the child's condition does not improve within one hour, consult a physician.

POSSIBLE SIDE EFFECTS
No serious side effects have been reported from the use of this product.

E-Mycin®

GENERIC NAME
Erythromycin.

PRODUCT CATEGORY
Antibiotic.

DOSAGE FORM
Tablets, enteric-coated tablets (250 mg) (to prevent release of the drug in the stomach before it reaches the small intestine), oral suspension.

WHY PRESCRIBED
E-Mycin, as well as other forms of erythromycin, is used to treat mild or moderate bacterial infections, especially when the child is known to be allergic to penicillin or when the bacteria do not respond to penicillin.

CHILDREN'S DOSAGE
This depends largely on the severity of the infection and the child's age and weight. The usual total daily dosage is 30 to 50 milligrams per kilogram of body weight (1 kilogram = 2.2 pounds), given in divided doses three or four times per day. In treating particularly severe infections the physician may double this amount.

PRECAUTIONS AND WARNINGS
Children should take E-Mycin at the times and in the exact amounts prescribed by their physicians. Taking more than the prescribed amount can result in such adverse effects as stomach discomfort, nausea, vomiting, and diarrhea.

Long-term use of any antibiotic may result in the development of a "superinfection"—the growth and multiplication in the body of fungi and other microorganisms that are not affected by the drug. Dispose of any remaining product once the course of therapy has been successfully completed.

The doctor should be advised if the child is taking other medications, such as theophylline or phenytoin products, that may cause an adverse reaction when taken with erythromycin.

POSSIBLE SIDE EFFECTS
E-Mycin, as well as most other forms of erythromycin, is a relatively safe antibiotic. Serious side effects are uncommon. Among reported side effects are digestive system upsets, including abdominal pain, nausea and vomiting, and diarrhea (because erythromycin may stimulate activity of the gastrointestinal tract); hypersensitivity (allergic) reactions marked by skin rashes and hives (urticaria), liver disorders with jaundice; and temporary loss of hearing, which may be due to the use of large doses.

Epifoam®

GENERIC NAME
This product contains a combination of hydrocortisone acetate (1 percent), cetylalcohol, and various other ingredients.

PRODUCT CATEGORY
Topical corticosteroid/anti-inflammatory/antipruritic (anti-itching).

DOSAGE FORM
Aerosol foam (pressurized container).

WHY PRESCRIBED
It is used for the relief of symptoms of inflammation and itching caused by certain skin diseases.

CHILDREN'S DOSAGE
This product is for external use only. It should not be applied to the skin of any child with a known sensitivity (allergy) to the ingredients. When applied to the diaper area of an infant, the child should not wear tight-fitting diapers or plastic pants that would form an airtight seal over the medicated skin. Only the minimum amount of the drug prescribed by the doctor should be applied to the affected skin of the child.

PRECAUTIONS AND WARNINGS
Because children tend to be more sensitive to the effects of corticosteroid drugs than adults, special care should be taken to avoid application of the product to large skin areas, prolonged or excessive application of the drug, or addition of an occlusive (air-tight) dressing over the treated skin area. The treated area should not be bandaged or otherwise covered or wrapped, except as directed by a physician. Any signs of an adverse skin reaction should be reported immediately to the doctor.

POSSIBLE SIDE EFFECTS
Among side effects reported from use of corticosteroid preparations applied to the skin are burning, itching, irritation, dryness, maceration (softening) of the skin, loss of skin color in the area treated, secondary infections, streaking of the skin, and miliaria (prickly heat).

ERYC®

GENERIC NAME
Erythromycin.

PRODUCT CATEGORY
Antibiotic.

DOSAGE FORM
Capsules (containing enteric-coated pellets to prevent release of the drug in the stomach before it reaches the small intestine).

WHY PRESCRIBED
It is used to treat mild to moderate bacterial infections of the upper and lower respiratory tracts, including whooping cough, conjunctivitis (inflammation of the membranes of the eyelids), and certain infections of the skin and digestive tract. It is frequently recommended as an alternative antibiotic for use in children who are allergic to penicillin-type drugs.

CHILDREN'S DOSAGE
This depends largely on the age and weight of the child and the severity of the infection. The usual recommended dosage is between 30 milligrams and 50 milligrams per kilogram of body weight (1 kilogram = 2.2 pounds) per day in divided doses. For a severe infection, the dosage may be doubled by the physician.

PRECAUTIONS AND WARNINGS
This product should not be given to children who are known to be hypersensitive (allergic) to the drug. Erythromycin preparations should not be given to a child with a liver disorder without the advice of a physician. The doctor also should be consulted about possible interactions between ERYC and other medications taken by the child, particularly theophylline medications prescribed for asthma or other respiratory disorders.

Long-term use of any antibiotic may result in the development of a "superinfection"—the growth and multiplication in the body of fungi and other microorganisms that are not affected by the drug.

POSSIBLE SIDE EFFECTS
The most frequently reported side effects of erythromycin drugs include skin rashes; urticaria (hives); eczema; digestive system symptoms of nausea, vomiting, diarrhea, loss of appetite, and abdominal pain; and temporary loss of hearing, usually due to the use of large doses.

EryPed®

GENERIC NAME
Erythromycin ethylsuccinate.

PRODUCT CATEGORY
Antibiotic.

DOSAGE FORM
Oral suspension (400 mg per 5 ml teaspoonful when reconstituted).

WHY PRESCRIBED
EryPed is used to treat mild to moderate bacterial infections, especially when the child is known to be allergic to penicillin or when the infection does not respond to penicillin. It is prescribed for treatment of bacterial infections of the upper respiratory tract, skin, urinary tract, digestive tract, and certain specific diseases.

CHILDREN'S DOSAGE
This depends largely on the age and weight of the child and the severity of the infection. For mild to moderate infections, the usual recommended dosage is between 30 and 50 milligrams per kilogram of body weight (1 kilogram = 2.2 pounds) per day in equally divided doses. For more severe infections, the dosage may be doubled by the physician.

PRECAUTIONS AND WARNINGS
EryPed should not be given to a child with a known hypersensitivity (allergy) to this antibiotic. Caution should be used in giving the drug to a child with a liver disorder. The doctor should be advised if the child is taking any other medication, particularly a theophylline product, which may interact unfavorably with the antibiotic.

Long-term use of any antibiotic may result in the development of a "superinfection"—the growth and multiplication in the body of fungi and other microorganisms that are not affected by the drug.

POSSIBLE SIDE EFFECTS
The most commonly reported side effects include digestive system disorders such as nausea, vomiting, diarrhea, and abdominal cramps. There also may be mild skin eruptions, including urticaria (hives), and temporary hearing impairment, particularly after taking large doses.

Erythrocin® Stearate

GENERIC NAME
Erythromycin stearate.

PRODUCT CATEGORY
Antibiotic.

DOSAGE FORM
Tablets (125 mg and 500 mg).

WHY PRESCRIBED
Erythrocin stearate, like other forms of erythromycin, is used to treat mild to moderate bacterial infections—especially when the child is known to be allergic to penicillin or when the bacteria do not respond to penicillin. It also may be prescribed to treat certain specific diseases.

CHILDREN'S DOSAGE
This depends largely on the severity of the infection and the child's age and weight. The usual total daily dosage is 30 to 50 milligrams per kilogram of body weight (1 kilogram = 2.2 pounds), given in divided doses three or four times per day. In treating severe infections, the physician may increase the dosage to double that amount.

PRECAUTIONS AND WARNINGS
This product should not be given to a child with a known hypersensitivity (allergy) to erythromycin antibiotics. Children should take Erythrocin stearate at the times and in the exact amounts prescribed by their physicians. Taking more than the prescribed amount increases the risk of adverse side effects. It should be used with caution in a child with liver impairment. The doctor should be advised if the child is taking another medication, particularly one containing theophylline, which may interact adversely with the antibiotic.

Long-term use of any antibiotic may result in the development of a "superinfection"—the growth of fungi and other microorganisms that are not affected by the drug.

POSSIBLE SIDE EFFECTS
The most commonly reported side effects involve digestive system complaints of nausea, vomiting, diarrhea, and abdominal cramps, usually due to the use of large doses of erythromycin (generic). Large doses also may result in temporary loss of hearing. Skin eruptions and urticaria (hives) also have been associated with the use of erythromycin products.

erythromycin (generic)

BRAND NAMES
E.E.S.®, E-Mycin®, ERYC®, EryPed®, Erythrocin® Stearate, Ethril®, Pediamycin®, SK-Erythromycin®, Wyamycin®.

PRODUCT CATEGORY
Antibiotic.

DOSAGE FORM
Tablets, chewable tablets, capsules, oral suspension, pediatric drops, skin ointment, and eye ointment.

WHY PRESCRIBED
Erythromycins are generally used to treat mild to moderate bacterial infections, especially when the child is known to be allergic to penicillin or when the bacteria are resistant to penicillin.

CHILDREN'S DOSAGE
The ointment forms of erythromycin should be used as directed by the physician. The dosage of the oral forms of the drug (to be taken by mouth) depends largely on the severity of the infection and the child's age and body weight. The usual total daily dosage is 30 milligrams to 50 milligrams per kilogram of body weight (1 kilogram = 2.2 pounds), given in equally divided doses three or four times per day. In treating particularly severe infections, the physician may double this amount.

PRECAUTIONS AND WARNINGS
Children should take erythromycin at the times and in the exact amounts prescribed by their physicians. Taking more than the prescribed amount is not only wasteful but may lead to adverse effects. Do not mix erythromycin drugs with other medications such as theophylline (used to treat asthma), without first consulting the doctor.

Long-term use of any antibiotic may result in the development of a "superinfection"—the growth and multiplication in the body of fungi and other microorganisms that are not affected by the drug.

POSSIBLE SIDE EFFECTS
Erythromycin is a relatively safe antibiotic and serious side effects are uncommon. However, erythromycin may cause skin rashes or hives (urticaria) in certain hypersensitive (allergic) individuals. The drug also has a tendency to stimulate gastrointestinal activity, resulting in abdominal cramps, nausea, vomiting, and diarrhea. It may affect the liver adversely, producing signs of jaundice. Large doses of the drug can result in a temporary loss of normal hearing.

Eurax®

GENERIC NAME
Crotamiton.

PRODUCT CATEGORY
Scabicide/antipruritic.

DOSAGE FORM
Cream and lotion.

WHY PRESCRIBED
It is used to eradicate scabies, a communicable skin disease caused by the itch mite (*Sarcoptes scabei*). Eurax is also effective in relieving general itching (pruritus).

CHILDREN'S DOSAGE
To treat scabies, both children and adults should take a bath or shower, then rub Eurax cream or lotion thoroughly into every skin area, from the chin to the toes. Apply again twenty-four hours later. Wash the medication off the skin about forty-eight hours after the final application. To prevent recontamination, clothing and bed linen should be dry-cleaned or washed in hot water.
As a treatment to relieve itching, massage Eurax into affected areas until it is absorbed. Repeat as required.

PRECAUTIONS AND WARNINGS
This product is for external use only. It should not be used on children who may have an allergic sensitivity to the product. Do not apply Eurax to raw or inflamed areas of skin. Keep the product away from the eyes or mouth.
Discontinue use of Eurax at the first sign of skin irritation or other evidence of an allergic reaction and consult a physician.

POSSIBLE SIDE EFFECTS
Some children may experience skin irritation or an allergic skin rash. The most serious adverse effect may result from accidental ingestion (swallowing) of the product by a child, which can result in a burning sensation in the mouth, irritation of the mouth and digestive tract, nausea, vomiting, and abdominal pain.

Feosol® (OTC)

GENERIC NAME
Ferrous sulfate.

PRODUCT CATEGORY
Elemental iron (dietary supplement).

DOSAGE FORM
Elixir, timed-release capsules, and tablets.

WHY USED
It is used in the treatment of children with a dietary or nutritional deficiency of iron (simple iron-deficiency anemia). This can occur, for example, in infants who are weaned relatively late from a milk diet, as milk is naturally deficient in iron. It may also occur in older children when rapid growth (with a corresponding increase in the volume of circulating blood) results in a need for more iron than can be absorbed from the child's diet.

CHILDREN'S DOSAGE
Even though this product is available without a doctor's prescription, a physician should be consulted before giving ferrous sulfate to a child. Giving excessive amounts of iron to children can be extremely dangerous. Follow the directions on the label carefully.

PRECAUTIONS AND WARNINGS
Infants and children should not be given dietary supplements of iron or products that contain iron without the advice and supervision of a physician. Only a physician can determine if a child has a true need for supplemental iron. Giving a child an excessive amount of iron can cause toxic symptoms and can even be fatal. *Never* give an adult dose to a child.

POSSIBLE SIDE EFFECTS
Some children taking iron supplements may experience nausea, abdominal pain, or constipation. The doctor may suggest that iron be taken with meals to minimize the gastrointestinal disturbances.

Fer-In-Sol® (OTC)

GENERIC NAME
Ferrous sulfate.

PRODUCT CATEGORY
Elemental iron (dietary supplement).

DOSAGE FORM
Syrup, capsules, and pediatric drops.

WHY USED
It is used in the treatment of children with a dietary or nutritional deficiency of iron (simple iron-deficiency anemia). This can occur, for example, in infants who are weaned relatively late from a milk diet, which is naturally deficient in iron. It may also occur in older children when rapid growth (with a corresponding increase in the volume of circulating blood) results in a need for more iron than can be absorbed from the child's diet.

CHILDREN'S DOSAGE
Although ferrous sulfate (iron) is available without a doctor's prescription, it is not recommended that children be given iron supplements without medical supervision. Giving excessive amounts of iron to children can be extremely dangerous. Follow the directions on the label.

PRECAUTIONS AND WARNINGS
Infants and children should not be given dietary supplements of iron or products that contain iron without the advice and supervision of a physician. Only a physician can determine if a child has a true need for supplemental iron. In addition, giving a child an excessive amount of iron can cause toxic symptoms and can even be fatal. *Never* give an adult dose to a child.

POSSIBLE SIDE EFFECTS
Some children taking iron supplements may experience nausea, abdominal pain, or constipation. The doctor may suggest that the iron be taken with meals to minimize the gastrointestinal disturbances.

Fero-Gradumet® (OTC)

GENERIC NAME
Ferrous sulfate.

PRODUCT CATEGORY
Elemental iron (dietary supplement).

DOSAGE FORM
Filmtab® timed-release tablets.

WHY USED
It is used in the treatment of children with a dietary or nutritional deficiency of iron (simple iron-deficiency anemia). This can occur, for example, in infants who are weaned relatively late from a milk diet, which is naturally deficient in iron. It may also occur in older children when rapid growth (with a corresponding increase in the volume of circulating blood) results in a need for more iron than can be absorbed from the child's diet.

CHILDREN'S DOSAGE
Even though ferrous sulfate (iron) is available without a doctor's prescription, it is not recommended that children be given iron supplements without medical supervision. Giving excessive amounts of iron to children can be dangerous. Follow the directions on the label.

PRECAUTIONS AND WARNINGS
Infants and children should not be given dietary supplements of iron or products that contain iron without the advice and supervision of a physician. Only a physician can determine if a child has a true need for supplemental iron. In addition, giving a child an excessive amount of iron can cause toxic symptoms and can even be fatal. *Never* give an adult dose to a child.

POSSIBLE SIDE EFFECTS
Some children taking iron supplements may experience nausea, abdominal pain, or constipation. The doctor may suggest that the iron be taken with meals to minimize the gastrointestinal disturbances.

ferrous sulfate (generic) (OTC)

BRAND NAMES
Feosol®, Fer-In-Sol®, Fero-Gradumet®, Mol-Iron®.

PRODUCT CATEGORY
Elemental iron (dietary supplement).

DOSAGE FORM
Elixir, syrup, liquid, tablets, and capsules.

WHY USED
It is used in the treatment of children with a dietary or nutritional deficiency of iron (simple iron-deficiency anemia). This can occur, for example, in infants who are weaned relatively late from a milk diet, which is naturally deficient in iron. It may also occur in older children when rapid growth (with a corresponding increase in the volume of circulating blood) results in a need for more iron than can be absorbed from the child's diet.

CHILDREN'S DOSAGE
Even though ferrous sulfate (iron) is available without a doctor's prescription, it should not be given to children without medical supervision. Giving excessive amounts of iron to children can be dangerous. Follow the directions on the label.

PRECAUTIONS AND WARNINGS
Infants and children should not be given dietary supplements of iron or products that contain iron without the advice and supervision of a physician. Only a physician can determine whether a child has a true need for supplemental iron. In addition, giving a child an excessive amount of iron can cause toxic symptoms and can even be fatal. *Never* give an adult dose to a child.

POSSIBLE SIDE EFFECTS
Some children taking iron supplements may experience nausea, abdominal pain, or constipation. The doctor may suggest that the iron be taken with meals to minimize the gastrointestinal disturbances.

Formula 44® Cough Mixture (OTC)

GENERIC NAME
This product contains in every dose of two teaspoonfuls (10 ml) a combination of dextromethorphan hydrobromide (30 mg), doxylamine succinate (7.5 mg), and alcohol (10 percent).

PRODUCT CATEGORY
Antitussive (cough suppressant)/antihistamine/demulcent (irritation reducer).

DOSAGE FORM
Syrup.

WHY USED
It is used to relieve the coughing associated with the common cold, flu, or bronchitis. The product also reduces sneezing and runny nose and coats and soothes the mucous membranes of the throat.

CHILDREN'S DOSAGE
This product should not be given to children under the age of six years without medical approval. The usual dosage for children between the ages of six and twelve years is one teaspoonful (5 ml) every four hours, up to a maximum of six teaspoonfuls a day. Children aged twelve years and over are usually given two teaspoonfuls (10 ml) every four hours, up to a maximum of six doses (12 teaspoonfuls) daily.

PRECAUTIONS AND WARNINGS
Do not exceed the dosage recommended by the child's physician. Prolonged coughing, especially if accompanied by a fever or headache, may indicate a serious medical problem. In such cases, stop giving the child any cough remedy and consult a physician. Use of the product also should be stopped and a doctor consulted if the symptoms are not relieved within three days.

POSSIBLE SIDE EFFECTS
The most common side effects include drowsiness, headache, nausea, vomiting, dizziness, and impaired muscular coordination (ataxia).

Furadantin®

GENERIC NAME
Nitrofurantoin.

PRODUCT CATEGORY
Antiseptic/antimicrobial (urinary tract).

DOSAGE FORM
Liquid (oral suspension) and tablets.

WHY PRESCRIBED
It is used in the treatment of bacterial infections of the urinary tract (when caused by susceptible strains of bacteria).

CHILDREN'S DOSAGE
This depends on the weight of the child. The usual total daily dosage is 5 to 7 milligrams per kilogram of body weight (1 kilogram = 2.2 pounds), given in divided doses four times daily.

PRECAUTIONS AND WARNINGS
Furadantin should not be given to children under the age of one month or to any child with a known hypersensitivity (allergy) to nitrofurantoin or related drugs. It also should not be given to children with impaired kidney function. The drug should be used with great caution (if at all) in children with impaired kidney function, diabetes, anemia, vitamin B deficiency, or any debilitating disease.

POSSIBLE SIDE EFFECTS
The most commonly reported side effects include loss of appetite (anorexia), nausea, vomiting, diarrhea, abdominal pain, and drug-induced fever.

Although more severe side effects are relatively uncommon, a few children taking Furadantin may experience potentially serious allergic (hypersensitivity) reactions. Among those reported are inflammation of the lungs (pneumonitis), inflammation of the liver (hepatitis), and a generalized severe allergic reaction (anaphylactic shock).

Gantanol®

GENERIC NAME
Sulfamethoxazole.

PRODUCT CATEGORY
Antibacterial (sulfonamide).

DOSAGE FORM
Liquid (oral suspension) and tablets.

WHY PRESCRIBED
It is used mainly to treat infants (over the age of two months) and children who have infections of the urinary tract (kidneys and bladder).

CHILDREN'S DOSAGE
This depends on the child's weight. The usual total daily dosage is 25 to 30 milligrams per kilogram of body weight (1 kilogram = 2.2 pounds), given in the morning and in the evening, following an initial dose that is twice the usual daily size. For example, a child weighing 18 kilograms (40 pounds) would be given a starting dose of two 500 mg tablets or two teaspoonfuls of Gantanol, after which the dosage would be one tablet or one teaspoonful in the morning and another in the evening each day for the course of the therapy.

PRECAUTIONS AND WARNINGS
Be sure the child drinks plenty of water or other fluids while taking Gantanol. This helps prevent the formation of crystals of the drug that could damage the kidneys.

Gantanol should be given with caution (if at all) to children with a disease of the kidneys or liver, severe allergies, or bronchial asthma.

POSSIBLE SIDE EFFECTS
The most commonly reported side effects are nausea, vomiting, dizziness, and headache. Some patients taking this class of antibacterial (a sulfa drug) may experience allergic (hypersensitivity) reactions, ranging from skin rashes to life-threatening anaphylactic shock.

Stop giving Gantanol to a child who develops skin rash, sore throat, or jaundice (yellowness of the skin), and consult a physician immediately.

Gantrisin® Pediatric Suspension and Syrup

GENERIC NAME
Acetyl sulfisoxazole.

PRODUCT CATEGORY
Antibacterial (sulfonamide).

DOSAGE FORM
Pediatric suspension and syrup; a long-acting Lipo form in vegetable oil is also available.

WHY PRESCRIBED
It is used mainly to treat susceptible bacterial infections of the urinary tract (kidneys and bladder).

CHILDREN'S DOSAGE
Gantrisin is not recommended for children under the age of two months, except with the advice and supervision of a physician. For older children, dosage depends on the child's weight. The usual daily dosage is 150 milligrams per kilogram of body weight (1 kilogram = 2.2 pounds), given in equally divided doses four times daily. For the very first dose, most physicians prescribe one-half of the total daily dose, or 75 milligrams per kilogram of body weight. If the Lipo Gantrisin form of the drug is used, the first dose for infants over the age of two months and children is 60 milligrams to 75 milligrams per kilogram of body weight, after which the child is given 60 to 75 milligrams per kilogram twice daily. When any of the liquid forms of Gantrisin are used (suspension, syrup or long-acting Lipo), the maximum total daily dose should not exceed 6 grams (6,000 milligrams), regardless of the weight of the child.

PRECAUTIONS AND WARNINGS
Gantrisin should be given with caution (if at all) to children with a disease of the kidneys or liver, severe allergies, or bronchial asthma.
  Be sure the child drinks plenty of water or other fluids while taking Gantrisin. This helps prevent the formation of crystals of the drug that could damage the kidneys.

POSSIBLE SIDE EFFECTS
The most commonly reported side effects are nausea, vomiting, dizziness, and headache. Some individuals given this class of antibacterial (a sulfa drug) may experience allergic or hypersensitivity reactions, ranging from skin rashes to life-threatening anaphylactic shock.
  Stop giving Gantrisin to a child who develops skin rashes, sore throat, or jaundice (yellowness of the skin), and consult a physician immediately.

Glycotuss® (OTC)

GENERIC NAME
Guaifenesin (100 mg per 5 ml teaspoonful or tablet).

PRODUCT CATEGORY
Expectorant.

DOSAGE FORM
Syrup and tablets.

WHY USED
This product is used to loosen phlegm (sputum) and bronchial secretions in the relief of symptoms of dry, unproductive coughs associated with the common cold, measles, pertussis (whooping cough), and influenza.

CHILDREN'S DOSAGE
This product is not recommended for use in children under the age of two years, unless directed by a physician.

Age of Child	Tablets or Teaspoonfuls (5 ml) Every Four Hours
2–6 years	½
6–12 years	1

The child should not receive more than six doses in any 24-hour period.

PRECAUTIONS AND WARNINGS
This product should not be given to any child with a known hypersensitivity to guaifenesin.

POSSIBLE SIDE EFFECTS
No serious side effects have been reported.

Indocin®

GENERIC NAME
Indomethacin.

PRODUCT CATEGORY
Anti-inflammatory (nonsteroidal).

DOSAGE FORM
Capsules (25 mg and 50 mg), oral suspension, in sustained-release (SR) capsules (75 mg), and suppositories (50 mg).

WHY PRESCRIBED
It is used to relieve the symptoms of pain and inflammation associated with a wide variety of severe joint disorders, including ankylosing spondylitis, osteoarthritis, and rheumatoid arthritis.

CHILDREN'S DOSAGE
Indocin is not generally recommended for use in children under the age of fourteen years. The dosage for older children (and adults) is determined by the physician. In all cases it should be the absolute minimum amount of the drug that will provide prompt relief of painful symptoms.

PRECAUTIONS AND WARNINGS
Indocin is an extremely potent drug with a potential for causing serious side effects. It should never be used casually or to treat conditions for which it is not intended. Parents should never "borrow" this drug to treat their own symptoms. It should *never* be taken without the knowledge of a physician.

POSSIBLE SIDE EFFECTS
The most commonly reported side effects include headache, nausea, vomiting, upset stomach, heartburn, and dizziness. Some patients also experience anxiety, mental confusion, blurred vision, high blood pressure (hypertension), chest pain, hearing disturbances, swelling of tissues (edema) caused by fluid retention, low blood pressure (hypotension), skin rashes, and impairment of the blood-forming tissues (which may, though rarely, lead to fatal complications).

Intal®

GENERIC NAME
Cromolyn sodium.

PRODUCT CATEGORY
Antiasthmatic/antiallergic.

DOSAGE FORM
Ampules of nebulizer solution (for inhalation).

WHY PRESCRIBED
It is used to prevent the symptoms of bronchial asthma, especially in children who may be hypersensitive (allergic) to the effects of other antiasthmatic drugs, such as theophylline.

CHILDREN'S DOSAGE
This product is not recommended for children under the age of two years. For older children (and adults), the contents of one ampule is administered by nebulization four times a day, usually through a face mask, at the start of therapy. The dosage may be adjusted downward later, depending on the needs and response of the child.

PRECAUTIONS AND WARNINGS
This drug should not be given to any child who has a known hypersensitivity (allergy) to cromolyn sodium products. It is not recommended for use in cases of acute asthma attacks or status asthmaticus. Caution should be used in giving the drug to a child with impaired kidney or liver function. Symptoms of asthma may recur if the dosage is reduced or discontinued.

POSSIBLE SIDE EFFECTS
Among side effects reported in persons using cromolyn sodium are nasal congestion, wheezing, sneezing, coughing, nasal itching, nosebleeds, stomach ache, and nausea.

ipecac syrup (generic) (OTC)

BRAND NAMES
This product is not marketed under a brand name.

PRODUCT CATEGORY
Emetic.

DOSAGE FORM
Syrup.

WHY USED
It is used to induce vomiting (emetic action) in the emergency treatment of certain cases of poisoning and drug overdosage.

CHILDREN'S DOSAGE
Ipecac syrup is available without a doctor's prescription. Administer to children only on the advice of a physician or a poison control center. The usual dosage for children one year of age and older is three teaspoonfuls (15 ml) followed by a glass of water. If vomiting does not occur within *twenty minutes*, a second dose may be tried. If vomiting does not occur within the next *ten minutes*, consult a physician at once.

PRECAUTIONS AND WARNINGS
Be extremely careful that you do NOT use ipecac *fluid extract* by mistake. It is fourteen times more potent than ipecac *syrup* and has caused deaths!

No emetic should ever be given to an unconscious person. If vomiting does not occur within thirty minutes of administering ipecac syrup, obtain immediate medical assistance.

Vomiting should *not* be induced if certain medications or chemicals are injested. Always consult a physician or a poison control center *before* using ipecac syrup.

Isopto Carpine®

GENERIC NAME
Pilocarpine hydrochloride.

PRODUCT CATEGORY
Ophthalmic (eye) preparation/antiglaucomat agent.

DOSAGE FORM
Eyedrops (solution).

WHY PRESCRIBED
It is used in the treatment of glaucoma, a disease characterized by abnormally high fluid pressure within the eyeball. Isopto Carpine causes a drop in this pressure, thereby relieving damaging pressure on the optic nerve.

CHILDREN'S DOSAGE
This depends on the severity of the condition and the child's response to Isopto Carpine therapy. The physician will determine the dosage based on individual need.

PRECAUTIONS AND WARNINGS
Do not let the dropper touch the eye while administering eyedrops. Do not allow the dropper to touch anything that might contaminate it.

Isopto Carpine should be used with caution in children with bronchial asthma or high blood pressure (hypertension).

Be sure to explain to the child that vision will be blurred temporarily after the drug is instilled in the eye.

POSSIBLE SIDE EFFECTS
Some children may experience local irritation or evidence of an allergic reaction. Should this occur, consult the doctor.

Kaopectate® (OTC)

GENERIC NAME
This product contains a combination of kaolin and pectin.

PRODUCT CATEGORY
Antidiarrheal.

DOSAGE FORM
Liquid (oral suspension) and tablets.

WHY USED
It is used to control common diarrhea.

CHILDREN'S DOSAGE
Kaopectate is available without a doctor's prescription. Administer to children exactly as the label recommends.

PRECAUTIONS AND WARNINGS
If the child has severe or prolonged diarrhea, consult a doctor at once so that a more serious underlying problem can be ruled out or diagnosed and treated. Do not give a child this product for more than two days or in the presence of a high fever.

Do not give Kaopectate to a child with heart disease, asthma, or other chronic illnesses without medical advice.

POSSIBLE SIDE EFFECTS
Used as directed, side effects are relatively infrequent.

Keflex®

GENERIC NAME
Cephalexin.

PRODUCT CATEGORY
Antibiotic (cephalosporin).

DOSAGE FORM
Oral suspension, capsules, and tablets.

WHY PRESCRIBED
It is used to treat certain bacterial infections that involve the respiratory tract, the skin and soft tissues, and the urinary tract, and some bone infections. Many physicians limit the use of Keflex to those infections that are especially susceptible to cephalosporin. Also, it may be prescribed when a child is known to be allergic to another antibiotic.

CHILDREN'S DOSAGE
This depends largely on the type of infection and the body weight of the child. For infections of the skin and throat, the usual total daily dosage is 25 to 50 milligrams per kilogram of body weight (1 kilogram = 2.2 pounds), given in divided doses according to the instructions of the physician. In cases of very severe infections, that dosage may be doubled by the physician. For otitis media (infection of the middle ear), the physician may prescribe daily dosages of 75 to 100 milligrams per kilogram of body weight, given in divided doses.

PRECAUTIONS AND WARNINGS
Children who are allergic to penicillin may also be allergic to Keflex. Thus, before administering this drug to such hypersensitive patients, they should be tested for possible allergic reactions. The child should also be closely monitored by the physician during the course of therapy. Special care is advised in giving the drug to a child with a kidney disorder.

POSSIBLE SIDE EFFECTS
The most commonly reported side effects include diarrhea, dizziness, vomiting, upset stomach, abdominal discomfort or pain, and skin rashes. A few patients taking this class of drugs have also experienced severe allergic reactions (anaphylactic shock).

Kenalog®

GENERIC NAME
Triamcinolone acetonide.

PRODUCT CATEGORY
Anti-inflammatory (synthetic corticosteroid).

DOSAGE FORM
Cream, lotion, ointment, spray (for direct application to affected areas of skin).

WHY PRESCRIBED
Kenalog is used to treat various inflammatory disorders of the skin that are responsive to corticosteroids.

CHILDREN'S DOSAGE
The physician will give specific directions for use. In general, ointment forms are used to treat dry or scaly areas of inflamed skin. Apply to the skin in a thin film two to four times daily. If the inflamed area is moist, the cream or lotion form of the drug should be used. Rub gently into the affected skin two or three times daily.

PRECAUTIONS AND WARNINGS
Do not apply Kenalog to areas of the child's skin that are infected. The drug has no beneficial effect on bacterial or fungal infections, and it may cause the disease to spread to nearby healthy areas of skin.

If Kenalog causes local irritation, or if the inflammation seems to worsen, discontinue use of the drug and consult the physician.

POSSIBLE SIDE EFFECTS
The most commonly reported side effects include itching, dry skin, skin eruptions, and a burning sensation at the site of drug application.

More serious side effects may occur if Kenalog is applied to extensive areas of skin and left on for prolonged periods. However, this is unlikely if the child is under close medical supervision and the physician's instructions are followed carefully.

Keralyt® Gel

GENERIC NAME
This product contains a combination of salicylic acid (6 percent), propylene glycol, alcohol (19.4 percent), hydroxypropycellulose, and water.

PRODUCT CATEGORY
Keratolytic (dead skin remover).

DOSAGE FORM
Gel.

WHY PRESCRIBED
It is used to aid in the removal of overgrowths of dead skin cells, including verrucae (warts), psoriasis scales, horny layers of the palms and soles, and keratosis pilaris (plugs of dead cells in skin follicles).

CHILDREN'S DOSAGE
The medication is usually applied to the affected skin area at bedtime, after first soaking the skin to be removed for five minutes with wet packs or in a bath. The product is washed off the following morning. In some cases, the procedure may have to be repeated to achieve removal of the unwanted dead skin layers. Unless the hands are being treated, they should be washed after applying the product.

PRECAUTIONS AND WARNINGS
Keralyt Gel is for external use only. This product should not be used on any child under the age of two years. It also should not be used on any child who is known to be hypersensitive (allergic) to salicylic acid or any of the other ingredients in the preparation. For children under the age of twelve years or those with a liver or kidney disorder, the area of skin treated should be limited and the patient observed closely for possible signs of salicylate toxicity (poisoning), which may include nausea, vomiting, dizziness, hearing difficulties, behavioral changes, diarrhea, or abnormal breathing. If such signs or symptoms occur, notify the doctor immediately; he may recommend discontinuing the drug and increasing the child's intake of fluids to help excrete the product more rapidly through the urine. Avoid getting the product in the eyes or in contact with the mucous membranes (such as those of the mouth or nostrils).

POSSIBLE SIDE EFFECTS
In addition to symptoms of salicylate toxicity (See PRECAUTIONS AND WARNINGS), there may be excessive redness and scaling of skin, particularly if the product is applied to areas with open skin sores. If the child is taking another medication, the doctor should be advised, as salicylic acid may interact adversely with several categories of drugs.

Kwell®

GENERIC NAME
Lindane (1 percent).

PRODUCT CATEGORY
Antiparasitic (parasiticide).

DOSAGE FORM
Cream, lotion, and shampoo.

WHY PRESCRIBED
It is used to kill the following skin parasites: *Sarcoptes scabiei* (scabies), *Pediculus capitis* (head louse), and *Phthirus pubis* (crab louse), and their eggs.

CHILDREN'S DOSAGE
This depends largely on the dosage form and the type of parasitic infection. All forms of Kwell should be used with considerable caution in infants and children, because they are especially susceptible to the toxicity of the drug (which penetrates the skin).

The shampoo form is best suited for the treatment of head lice. Apply just enough to wet the child's hair and adjacent areas of the skin, taking care not to come near the eyes. Add enough water to form a good lather and work this into the hair. Allow lather to remain for four minutes, then rinse hair thoroughly, and towel dry. Remove any remaining nits with a fine-tooth comb or tweezers. Unless living lice are found seven days later, further treatment is not necessary.

Follow the directions of the physician for the use of the cream and lotion forms of Kwell.

PRECAUTIONS AND WARNINGS
Lindane penetrates human skin and can cause adverse effects on the central nervous system. Seizures have been reported after the use of lindane, although a direct cause has not been found. Simultaneous use of more than one form of Kwell may increase the risk of side effects. Kwell in any of its forms should never be used routinely or used as a regular shampoo. Doing so adds to the risk of local irritation and more serious side effects.

Administer Kwell to children exactly as directed by the physician. If the product accidentally gets in the eyes, flush them with water immediately.

POSSIBLE SIDE EFFECTS
Some children may experience skin irritation or eruptions at the site where Kwell is applied. Itching may persist after treatment has been successfully completed.

If Kwell is misused or left on the skin too long, it may cause potentially serious side effects, including disorders of the central nervous system and impairment of liver function.

Librax®

GENERIC NAME
This product is a combination of chlordiazepoxide hydrochloride (5 mg) and clidinium bromide (2.5 mg).

PRODUCT CATEGORY
Antispasmodic/minor tranquilizer.

DOSAGE FORM
Capsules.

WHY PRESCRIBED
It is used to reduce the frequency and severity of painful spasms of the stomach and intestines that are associated with various disorders of the gastrointestinal tract. Librax also helps relieve any anxiety the child may have about the condition.

CHILDREN'S DOSAGE
This depends on the severity of the symptoms and the child's response to Librax therapy. The physician will adjust the dosage to meet the needs of the individual patient.

PRECAUTIONS AND WARNINGS
Do not suddenly stop giving the child Librax without the knowledge and advice of the physician. Otherwise, the child may experience anxiety, insomnia, and nightmares.

POSSIBLE SIDE EFFECTS
The most commonly reported side effects include drowsiness, impaired coordination, confusion, blurred vision, dryness of the mouth, difficulty urinating, and nausea.

Lidex®

GENERIC NAME
Fluocinonide.

PRODUCT CATEGORY
Anti-inflammatory (synthetic corticosteroid).

DOSAGE FORM
Cream, gel, solution, and ointment.

WHY PRESCRIBED
It is used to treat various inflammatory disorders of the skin that are responsive to corticosteroids.

CHILDREN'S DOSAGE
The physician will give specific instructions for use. In general, the ointment form is used to treat dry or scaly areas of inflamed skin. The cream form should be used if the inflamed area is moist. Rub gently into the affected skin three or four times daily, as required.

PRECAUTIONS AND WARNINGS
Do not apply Lidex to areas of the child's skin that may be infected. The drug has no beneficial effect on bacterial or fungal infections, and it may cause the disease to spread to nearby healthy areas of the skin.

If Lidex causes local irritation, or if the inflammation seems to worsen, discontinue the use of the drug and consult the physician.

POSSIBLE SIDE EFFECTS
The most commonly reported side effects include itching, dry skin, skin eruptions, and a burning sensation at the site of drug application.

More serious side effects may occur if Lidex is applied to large areas of the skin and is left on for prolonged periods. However, this is unlikely if the child is under close medical supervision and the physician's instructions are followed carefully.

Liquiprin® (OTC)

GENERIC NAME
Acetaminophen (80 mg per 1.67 ml dropperful).

PRODUCT CATEGORY
Analgesic (pain reliever)/antipyretic (fever reducer).

DOSAGE FORM
Oral solution (raspberry flavor).

WHY USED
It is used to relieve symptoms of fever and pain associated with the common cold, flu, tonsillitis, teething, muscular aches, headache, digestive disorders, and immunization effects. It is an alternative choice for children who cannot tolerate aspirin products.

CHILDREN'S DOSAGE
The usual recommended dosage depends upon the age of the child, according to the following schedule:

Age of Child	Dropperfuls (80 mg at top mark)
Under 3 years	2
3 years	2
4–5 years	3

The doses can be repeated at four-hour intervals three to four times daily.

PRECAUTIONS AND WARNINGS
The drug should not be given to a child who is known to be hypersensitive (allergic) to acetaminophen. If a hypersensitivity reaction occurs, discontinue use of the drug and contact a physician.

POSSIBLE SIDE EFFECTS
Acetaminophen products are relatively free of side effects. In some children there may be a skin rash or urticaria (hives); digestive complaints, including nausea, vomiting, and abdominal pain; sweating; anemia and kidney and liver disorders. Most serious side effects are due to the use of large doses of the drug.

Lomotil®

GENERIC NAME
This product contains a combination of diphenoxylate hydrochloride (2.5 mg) and atropine sulfate (0.025 mg) in each tablet or 5 ml teaspoonful.

PRODUCT CATEGORY
Antidiarrheal.

DOSAGE FORM
Liquid and tablets.

WHY PRESCRIBED
It is used in the treatment of diarrhea. The mechanism of action is to slow down the peristaltic movements of the intestines.

CHILDREN'S DOSAGE
Lomotil should be given only in the *liquid* form to children between the ages of two and twelve years. The drug must not be given to children under the age of two years. The usual initial dosage is 0.3 to 0.4 milligrams per kilogram of body weight (1 kilogram = 2.2 pounds), given in divided doses. The physician will prescribe the exact dose (which may range, for example, from ½ to 1 teaspoonful four times daily for a six- to eight-year-old child weighing between 38 and 71 pounds). The doses are measured with a plastic dropper. The physician may reduce the dosage once the symptoms are under control. However, if no improvement is seen after forty-eight hours, the drug is unlikely to be effective.

PRECAUTIONS AND WARNINGS
Lomotil is an extremely potent drug. Giving a child more than the prescribed amounts can be dangerous. Children below the age of thirteen should receive only the liquid form of the product. If the diarrhea is not controlled within two days, consult the physician immediately. The excessive loss of body fluids in young children can cause potentially fatal dehydration.

POSSIBLE SIDE EFFECTS
The most commonly reported side effects include dry mouth, dry skin, difficulty urinating, flushing, rapid heartbeat (tachycardia), dizziness, nausea, vomiting, drowsiness, itching, and abdominal discomfort.

Lotrimin®

GENERIC NAME
Clotrimazole (1 percent).

PRODUCT CATEGORY
Antifungal.

DOSAGE FORM
Cream, lotion and solution (for direct application to the skin).

WHY PRESCRIBED
It is used to treat fungal infections of the skin, including tinea pedis (athlete's foot) and tinea corporis (ringworm of the body).

CHILDREN'S DOSAGE
Gently rub Lotrimin into the affected areas of the skin twice daily, in the morning and just before the child goes to bed. Improvement, including relief of itching, is usually noted after about one week.

PRECAUTIONS AND WARNINGS
Consult the child's physician if no improvement is seen after four weeks. The original diagnosis may have to be reviewed.

Do not apply a tight (occlusive) dressing over the treated skin area, unless you are advised to do so by the physician.

Take care not to get Lotrimin in or near the child's eyes.

POSSIBLE SIDE EFFECTS
Some children may develop a skin irritation or allergic reaction at the site of drug application. Other reported side effects include redness, peeling, swelling, itching, and hives (urticaria). Should any of these occur, consult the physician for advice about whether the use of Lotrimin should be discontinued.

Lytren® (OTC)

GENERIC NAME
This product contains a combination of water, corn syrup, dextrose, sodium citrate, potassium chloride, sodium biphosphate, potassium citrate, calcium chloride, and magnesium sulfate.

PRODUCT CATEGORY
Electrolyte replacement.

DOSAGE FORM
Liquid.

WHY USED
Lytren is used to provide vital minerals, carbohydrates, and fluids when the usual intake of foods and liquids has been discontinued, postsurgery, for example, or to supply fluid and nutrients in cases of mild to moderate diarrhea.

CHILDREN'S DOSAGE
The physician will prescribe the amount of Lytren to be given infants and young children, based on body surface area and replacement of fluid losses. For children between five and ten years of age, the usual recommended dosage is one to two quarts per day. For older children, the dosage may be two to three quarts per day. The prescribed dosage may be given in divided doses throughout the day. No more than the prescribed amount of Lytren should be given the child. If additional fluid is needed to satisfy thirst, it should be in the form of water or liquids, such as milk or fruit juices that do not contain electrolytes or mineral additives.

PRECAUTIONS AND WARNINGS
Lytren should not be given in the treatment of severe or continuing diarrhea or vomiting, when kidney function is impaired, or when the child has a serious gastrointestinal disorder such as a perforated bowel or an intestinal obstruction. The child should be given only the prescribed amount of Lytren. The product should not be mixed with or given with other liquids containing electrolytes, such as milk or fruit juices. Caution should be used in giving Lytren to a child who is also receiving water or electrolytes by intravenous feeding. Use of Lytren should be discontinued when normal feeding is resumed.

POSSIBLE SIDE EFFECTS
No serious side effects are expected when Lytren is used according to directions and under the supervision of a physician. Adverse effects of electrolyte imbalance may result when excessive or insufficient amounts of fluids or electrolytes are administered.

Macrodantin®

GENERIC NAME
Nitrofurantoin macrocrystals.

PRODUCT CATEGORY
Antimicrobial (urinary tract)/antiseptic.

DOSAGE FORM
Capsules.

WHY PRESCRIBED
It is used in the treatment of bacterial infections of the urinary tract caused by susceptible strains of bacteria.

CHILDREN'S DOSAGE
This depends on the weight of the child. The usual total daily dosage is 5 milligrams to 7 milligrams per kilogram of body weight (1 kilogram = 2.2 pounds), given in divided doses four times daily. It may be given with food or milk to minimize stomach upset.

PRECAUTIONS AND WARNINGS
Macrodantin should not be given to children under the age of one month. It should also not be given to children with impaired kidney function. The drug should be used with great caution (if at all) in children with diabetes, anemia, vitamin B deficiency, or any debilitating illness.

POSSIBLE SIDE EFFECTS
The most commonly reported side effects include loss of appetite (anorexia), nausea, vomiting, diarrhea, abdominal pain, and drug-induced fever.

Although more severe side effects are relatively uncommon, some patients taking Macrodantin may experience serious allergic reactions. Among these are inflammation of the lungs (pneumonitis), inflammation of the liver (hepatitis), and a generalized severe hypersensitivity reaction (anaphylactic shock).

Maltsupex® (OTC)

GENERIC NAME
Malt soup extract (nondiastatic extract from barley malt).

PRODUCT CATEGORY
Laxative.

DOSAGE FORM
Powder (to be mixed with warm water), liquid, and tablets.

WHY USED
It is used in infants and children to relieve simple constipation that is not related to a disease or disorder of the digestive tract.

CHILDREN'S DOSAGE
Maltsupex is available without a doctor's prescription. Administer to infants and children exactly as the label recommends. Be sure to give the child an adequate amount of fluid, such as water or fruit juice, with each dose.

PRECAUTIONS AND WARNINGS
Do not give a child any laxative in the presence of abdominal pain, high fever or nausea and vomiting. In such cases, consult a physician at once.

Consult a physician before giving Maltsupex to children with kidney disease.

The tablet form of Maltsupex contains an artificial coloring (tartrazine, or FD&C Yellow No. 5) that can cause attacks of bronchial asthma in susceptible children, especially those who are also allergic to aspirin, a related chemical.

The overuse or misuse of laxatimes can aggravate constipation or even cause the condition where it did not previously exist. Do not give a child laxatives regularly for more than one or two weeks without seeking medical advice. Although it is rare, the problem may be related to partial obstruction of the intestines and demand prompt medical diagnosis and treatment.

Constipation of infants is often related to dietary habits, such as ingesting large amounts of milk.

POSSIBLE SIDE EFFECTS
Maltsupex is a gentle laxative and, except for the tablet form, is relatively free from side effects. The dye in the tablets can cause asthmatic attacks in susceptible children.

Marax®

GENERIC NAME
Each tablet contains a combination of ephedrine sulfate (25 mg), theophylline (130 mg), and hydroxyzine hydrochloride (10 mg). (Each tablet is equivalent to four 5 ml teaspoonfuls of the syrup.)

PRODUCT CATEGORY
Bronchodilator/antiasthmatic.

DOSAGE FORM
Tablets and syrup.

WHY PRESCRIBED
It helps relieve wheezing and shortness of breath in children with bronchial asthma.

CHILDREN'S DOSAGE
Marax tablets should not be should not be given to children under the age of five years, or Marax syrup given to children under the age of two years. The physician will individualize the dosage depending on the severity of the condition and the response of the child to Marax therapy.

PRECAUTIONS AND WARNINGS
Do not give the child any other drugs at the same time as Marax without the knowledge and approval of the physician. Do not give this product to children with heart disease, thyroid disease, or high blood pressure (hypertension).

POSSIBLE SIDE EFFECTS
The most commonly reported side effects include drowsiness, rapid heartbeat (tachycardia), high blood pressure (hypertension), sensation of heartbeat (palpitations), headache, flushing, and dryness of the nose and throat. Some children taking Marax may also experience nausea, vomiting, and abdominal discomfort, particularly if the drug is taken on an empty stomach.

Marezine® (OTC)

GENERIC NAME
Cyclizine hydrochloride.

PRODUCT CATEGORY
Antiemetic/antihistamine.

DOSAGE FORM
Tablets.

WHY USED
It is used for the prevention or control of the symptoms of motion sickness, including nausea, vomiting, and dizziness.

CHILDREN'S DOSAGE
Marezine is available without a doctor's prescription. It should not be given to a child under the age of six years without the advice and supervision of a physician. Administer to children exactly as the label recommends.

PRECAUTIONS AND WARNINGS
Marezine should not be given to a child with a known allergic reaction to the drug. It should not be given to a child with glaucoma, except with the advice of a physician.

POSSIBLE SIDE EFFECTS
The most commonly reported side effect is drowsiness. Less frequently reported side effects include headache, dryness of the mouth and nose, diarrhea, and constipation.

Medrol®

GENERIC NAME
Methylprednisolone.

PRODUCT CATEGORY
Corticosteroid (synthetic glucocorticoid).

DOSAGE FORM
Tablets (it is also available as the acetate form in an ointment for external use only).

WHY PRESCRIBED
It is used in the treatment of a wide variety of inflammatory diseases of the skin, rheumatic disorders (such as juvenile rheumatoid arthritis, psoriatic arthritis, and ankylosing spondylitis), collagen diseases (including systemic lupus erythmatosus), allergies (including bronchial asthma and contact dermatitis), lung diseases, certain blood diseases, and other conditions.

Medrol is often used in combination with other corticosteroids in treating disorders of the adrenal glands, to replace hormones normally produced by these glands.

CHILDREN'S DOSAGE
This depends on the type and severity of the condition being treated and the response of the child to Medrol therapy. The physician will individualize the dosage to the child's requirements. In general, the lowest possible dose of corticosteroid drugs should be used and when a reduction in dosage is made, the reduction should be gradual.

PRECAUTIONS AND WARNINGS
Children should not be vaccinated against smallpox or be subjected to other immunization procedures while undergoing corticosteroid therapy. Because Medrol may interact with aspirin and many other prescription and nonprescription drugs, resulting in adverse effects, the doctor should be consulted about giving the child any additional medications while taking this product. Prednisone products may affect a child's response surgery, injury, or illness for up to two years after the drug has been discontinued. Thus, any doctor providing care for the child in the next two years should be advised of the child's previous use of the drug.

POSSIBLE SIDE EFFECTS
All drugs in the general class of corticosteroids, such as Medrol, are capable of causing a wide range of adverse effects. These are largely related to the dosage and the duration of the therapy. Among the reported side effects are suppressed growth; accumulation of fatty deposits around the face, neck, and abdomen; nervousness; a loss of density in bone tissue; increased susceptibility to infections; water retention, resulting in a swelling of the tissues (edema); euphoria; insomnia; skin changes; and increased susceptibility to bruising.

Meticorten®

GENERIC NAME
Prednisone.

PRODUCT CATEGORY
Corticosteroid (synthetic glucocorticoid)/anti-inflammatory.

DOSAGE FORM
Tablets.

WHY PRESCRIBED
It is used in the treatment of a wide variety of inflammatory and allergic conditions. Meticorten is often used in combination with other corticosteroids in treating disorders of the adrenal glands, to replace hormones normally produced by these glands.

CHILDREN'S DOSAGE
This depends on the type and severity of the condition being treated and the response of the child to Meticorten therapy. The physician will individualize the dosage to the child's requirements.

PRECAUTIONS AND WARNINGS
Children should not be vaccinated against smallpox or be subjected to other immunization procedures while undergoing corticosteroid therapy. Because Meticorten may interact with aspirin and many other prescription and nonprescription drugs, resulting in adverse effects, the doctor should be consulted about giving the child any additional medications while taking this product. Prednisone products may affect a child's response surgery, injury, or illness for up to two years after the drug has been discontinued. Thus, any doctor providing care for the child in the next two years should be advised of the child's previous use of the drug.

POSSIBLE SIDE EFFECTS
All drugs in the general class of corticosteroids, such as Meticorten, are capable of causing a wide range of adverse effects. These are largely related to the dosage and the duration of therapy. Among the reported side effects are suppressed growth in children; accumulation of fatty deposits around the face, neck, or abdomen; nervousness; a loss of bone tissue density (osteoporosis); increased susceptibility to infections; water retention resulting in a swelling of tissues (edema); euphoria; insomnia; skin changes; and increased susceptibility to bruising.

Metamucil® (OTC)

GENERIC NAME
Psyllium hydrophilic mucilloid.

PRODUCT CATEGORY
Laxative.

DOSAGE FORM
Powder (to be mixed with water).

WHY USED
It is used to relieve chronic constipation. Metamucil is known as a bulk laxative and contains dietary fiber from the husk of the psyllium seed (*Plantago ovata*). It closely approximates the physiological mechanism in promoting evacuation of the bowels.

CHILDREN'S DOSAGE
Metamucil is available without a doctor's prescription. Administer to children exactly as the label recommends.

PRECAUTIONS AND WARNINGS
Do not give a child Metamucil, or any laxative, in the presence of abdominal pain, high fever, or nausea and vomiting. In such cases, consult a physician at once.

The overuse of laxatives can aggravate constipation or even create the condition where it did not previously exist. Do not give a child laxatives regularly for more than one or two weeks without seeking medical advice. Although it is rare, the problem may be related to partial obstruction of the intestines and demand prompt medical diagnosis and treatment.

Constipation in infants is often related to dietary habits, such as ingesting large amounts of milk.

POSSIBLE SIDE EFFECTS
Metamucil is a gentle laxative and relatively free from side effects.

mineral oil (generic) (OTC)

BRAND NAMES
This product is not marketed under a brand name.

PRODUCT CATEGORY
Laxative.

DOSAGE FORM
Liquid.

WHY USED
It is used to lubricate the intestine in children who are constipated, thus helping reduce straining during bowel movements.

CHILDREN'S DOSAGE
The usual dosage is to give the child one tablespoonful (15 ml) in the morning and another at night (an additional tablespoonful may be given midday) until loose bowel movements occur four or five times a day. If significant improvement is not noted within one or two weeks, consult a physician.

PRECAUTIONS AND WARNINGS
Do not give a child any laxative in the presence of abdominal pain, high fever, or nausea and vomiting. In such cases, consult a physician at once.

The overuse of laxatives can aggravate constipation or even create the condition where it did not previously exist. Do not give the child laxatives regularly for more than one or two weeks without seeking medical advice. Although it is rare, the problem may be related to partial obstruction of the intestines and demand prompt medical diagnosis and treatment.

Constipation in infants is often related to dietary habits, such as drinking large amounts of milk.

POSSIBLE SIDE EFFECTS
Mineral oil is a gentle laxative and is relatively free from serious side effects. Laxatives may interfere with the absorption of medicines or nutrients, either by causing them to pass through the digestive tract too rapidly or by binding with them so that they are excreted rather than absorbed, thereby indirectly producing side effects.

Minocin®

GENERIC NAME
Minocycline hydrochloride (semisynthetic tetracycline).

PRODUCT CATEGORY
Antibacterial/antiamebic/antirickettsial.

DOSAGE FORM
Capsules, oral suspension, and tablets.

WHY PRESCRIBED
It is used to treat infections caused by a wide range of microorganisms, including certain species of bacteria, protozoa, and rickettsia (organisms between bacteria and viruses in size).

CHILDREN'S DOSAGE
This depends on the child's weight. The initial dosage for children over the age of eight is four milligrams per kilogram of body weight (1 kilogram = 2.2 pounds), followed by two milligrams per kilogram of body weight every twelve hours. Minocen should not be given to children under the age of eight, unless the physician determines that other antibiotics would be ineffective or inappropriate.

PRECAUTIONS AND WARNINGS
Tetracyclines may cause permanent discoloration of the teeth if given to children under the age of eight.

Do not give the child antacids while he or she is being treated with tetracycline, since this could interfere with the effectiveness of the antibiotic.

Tetracyclines should be used with caution (if at all) in children with impaired liver or kidney function.

POSSIBLE SIDE EFFECTS
The most common side effects include nausea, vomiting, diarrhea, heartburn, flatulence (intestinal gas), and loss of appetite (anorexia). Tetracyclines may cause potentially more serious side effects in some patients, including damage to the blood-forming tissues and severe generalized allergic reactions (anaphylactic shock).

Some children taking Minocin may experience severe skin eruptions and rashes when exposed to strong sunlight. These exaggerated "sunburn reactions" usually disappear days or weeks after therapy with tetracycline has been discontinued.

Monistat® 7 Vaginal Cream

GENERIC NAME
Miconazole nitrate.

PRODUCT CATEGORY
Antifungal agent.

DOSAGE FORM
Vaginal cream.

WHY PRESCRIBED
It is used to treat a specific local fungal infection (candidiasis) that affects the female external genitals and vagina. (Such infections in young girls are relatively uncommon.)

CHILDREN'S DOSAGE
The usual dosage is one applicatorful of Monistat (inserted into the vagina) once daily at bedtime. This is continued for seven days.

PRECAUTIONS AND WARNINGS
Stop giving the child Monistat at the first sign of local irritation or inflammation and consult the physician.

POSSIBLE SIDE EFFECTS
The most common side effects are a burning or itching sensation and irritation of the external genitals (vulva) or vagina. Some girls may also experience pelvic cramps, headaches, or skin rashes.

Motrin®

GENERIC NAME
Ibuprofen.

PRODUCT CATEGORY
Analgesic (pain reliever)/anti-inflammatory (nonsteroidal).

DOSAGE FORM
Tablets.

WHY PRESCRIBED
It is used to control the pain and inflammation of rheumatoid arthritis and osteoarthritis. It is also used to relieve the symptoms of mild to moderate pain and discomfort associated with dental procedures, minor surgery, or other disorders, including sports injuries.

CHILDREN'S DOSAGE
This product is available in strengths ranging from 400 to 800 milligrams, to be administered in dosages that are tailored for the individual according to the cause and severity of the pain and inflammation. The maximum daily dosage is 3,200 milligrams and is usually prescribed only for the severe pain of rheumatoid arthritis; the dosage for mild to moderate pain may be 1,600 to 2,400 milligrams per day, in divided doses.

PRECAUTIONS AND WARNINGS
Because ibuprofen suppresses symptoms of pain and inflammation, its use may conceal signs of complications or other serious disorders. It should not be given to a child who has shown a hypersensitivity (allergy) to this drug or to aspirin. It should not be given to children with certain disorders of the digestive tract, because ibuprofen may be a cause of peptic ulcers and gastrointestinal bleeding. It may also be a cause of edema (fluid retention and swollen tissues) and should be used with caution in children with high blood pressure or heart disease. Use of the drug should be discontinued if eye disorders such as blurred vision or changes in color vision occur.

POSSIBLE SIDE EFFECTS
The most commonly reported side effects are those involving the digestive tract, including nausea and vomiting, heartburn, abdominal pain, bloating and flatulence (gas), constipation, and diarrhea. Other side effects may include loss of appetite, skin rashes, dizziness, headaches, tinnitus (ringing in the ears), and nervousness.

Mycelex®

GENERIC NAME
Clotrimazole.

PRODUCT CATEGORY
Antifungal.

DOSAGE FORM
Troches (lozenges).

WHY PRESCRIBED
It is used in the treatment of candidiasis infections, caused by a yeast (*Candida albicans*), in the mouth and throat. The condition is also known as "thrush."

CHILDREN'S DOSAGE
The usual recommended dosage is one troche given by mouth and allowed to dissolve slowly, the dose being given five times a day for fourteen days.

PRECAUTIONS AND WARNINGS
Mycelex troches should not be given to a child who is known to be hypersensitive (allergic) to clotrimazole. The product is not recommended for other types of fungal infections. The product should not be given to a child who is not old enough to hold the troche in the mouth and allow it to dissolve slowly. It should not be given to a child with a liver disorder without the advice of a doctor.

POSSIBLE SIDE EFFECTS
The most commonly reported side effect is abnormal liver function. Other side effects are nausea and vomiting.

Mycelex® -G

GENERIC NAME
Clotrimazole.

PRODUCT CATEGORY
Antifungal.

DOSAGE FORM
Vaginal cream, and vaginal tablets.

WHY PRESCRIBED
This product is used in the treatment of yeast infections, particularly those caused by species of *Candida* in the female genital area, including the vagina.

CHILDREN'S DOSAGE
The usual recommended dosage for the tablets is one tablet a day, inserted into the vagina with a special applicator, once a day for seven days. The cream form of Mycelex-G is administered as one applicatorful (approximately 5 grams) inserted into the vagina each day for fourteen days. The drug is usually administered at bedtime.

PRECAUTIONS AND WARNINGS
The product should not be administered to a child who is known to be hypersensitive to clotrimazole or other ingredients included in the preparation. As Mycelex-G is effective only against vulvovaginal infections involving *Candida albicans* or related species of the yeast, it should not be used to treat other disorders of the female genital area.

POSSIBLE SIDE EFFECTS
Among reported side effects are a mild burning sensation, irritation, skin rash, increased frequency in the urge to urinate, and lower abdominal cramps.

Mycolog® II

GENERIC NAME
This product contains a combination of nystatin and triamcinolone acetonide.

PRODUCT CATEGORY
Antifungal/anti-inflammatory.

DOSAGE FORM
Cream and ointment.

WHY PRESCRIBED
It is used in the treatment of symptoms of redness and itching caused by skin infections by species of *Candida* yeasts, particularly *Candida albicans*.

CHILDREN'S DOSAGE
A thin film of the cream or ointment is applied to the affected skin area twice daily, in the morning and evening. Do not apply the drug to large areas of the skin. The cream form of the drug can be gently massaged into the skin. Use of either form of the drug should be discontinued if the symptoms persist for more than 25 days.

PRECAUTIONS AND WARNINGS
Mycolog II should not be used if the child is known to be hypersensitive (allergic) to the ingredients in the product. Discontinue giving the child Mycolog II if local irritation of the skin develops, and consult the physician. The drug should not be used for any disorder other than the condition for which it was prescribed. The treated area should not be bandaged or otherwise covered or wrapped tightly; when Mycolog II is used on the diaper area of infants, the child should not wear tightly fitting diapers or plastic pants. The risk of side effects is increased by using too much Mycolog II cream or ointment, treating an excessive area of skin, or covering the treated area with tightly fitting dressings or clothing.

POSSIBLE SIDE EFFECTS
Among reported side effects are burning, itching, dry skin, irritation, acnelike skin eruptions, changes in skin pigmentation, skin streaks, and miliaria (prickly heat).

Naldecon-DX® Pediatric Syrup (OTC)

GENERIC NAME
This product contains in each teaspoonful (5 ml) dextromethorphan hydrobromide (7.5 mg), phenylpropanolamine hydrochloride (9 mg), guaifenesin (100 mg), and alcohol (5 percent), and various other ingredients, including colorings and flavorings.

PRODUCT CATEGORY
Antitussive (cough suppressant)/decongestant/expectorant.

DOSAGE FORM
Pediatric syrup.

WHY USED
It is used to relieve coughing and nasal congestion (stuffy nose) associated with such conditions as bronchitis and the common cold. This product contains no antihistamines.

CHILDREN'S DOSAGE
This product is not recommend for use in children under the age of two years without the advice and supervision of a physician. The usual dosage for children between two and six years is one teaspoonful (5 ml) every four hours. Children over the age of six years may be given two teaspoonfuls every four hours. Do not give more than four doses in any 24-hour period.

PRECAUTIONS AND WARNINGS
This product should not be given to a child who has a known hypersensitivity (allergy) to any of the ingredients. It also should not be given to children who have asthma, diabetes, high blood pressure (hypertension), heart disorders, or thyroid disease without the knowledge and advice of a physician.

If the child's cough persists for more than one week, tends to recur, or is accompanied by a high fever or skin rash, stop giving the drug and consult a physician at once. These could be signs of a more serious underlying condition that requires prompt diagnosis and treatment.

POSSIBLE SIDE EFFECTS
Side effects, which include nervousness, dizziness, or sleeplessness, are usually related to giving the child more than the recommended dosage.

Naldecon-EX® Pediatric Drops (OTC)

GENERIC NAME
This product contains in each dropperful (1 ml) phenylpropanolamine hydrochloride (9 mg), guaifenesin (30 mg), and alcohol (0.6 percent).

PRODUCT CATEGORY
Decongestant/expectorant.

DOSAGE FORM
Pediatric drops.

WHY USED
Naldecon-EX Pediatric Drops are used to relieve nasal congestion (stuffy nose) and help loosen phlegm and mucus in the air passages, so they can be coughed up and expelled. The product is useful in conditions such as acute bronchitis, croup, and the common cold.

CHILDREN'S DOSAGE
Naldecon-EX Pediatric Drops are available without a doctor's prescription. However, the manufacturer cautions that this drug should not be given to children under the age of two years without medical advice. Administer to children over the age of two exactly as directed on the label.

PRECAUTIONS AND WARNINGS
This product should not be given to a child with a known hypersensitivity (allergy) to any of the ingredients. Do not give this product to children who have asthma, diabetes, high blood pressure (hypertension), heart disease, or thyroid disease without the knowledge and advice of a physician.

If the child's cough persists for more than one week, tends to recur, or is accompanied by a high fever or skin rash, stop giving the drug and consult a physician at once. These could be signs of a more serious underlying condition that requires prompt diagnosis and treatment.

POSSIBLE SIDE EFFECTS
Among reported side effects are nervousness, dizziness, and sleeplessness, which are usually related to giving the child more than the recommended dosage.

Neosporin® Ophthalmic Solution

GENERIC NAME
This product contains a combination of polymyxin B sulfate, neomycin sulfate, and gramicidin.

PRODUCT CATEGORY
Ophthalmic (eye) preparation/antibiotic.

DOSAGE FORM
Eyedrops.

WHY PRESCRIBED
It is used in the treatment of susceptible bacterial infections of the eye.

CHILDREN'S DOSAGE
This depends on the severity of the infection. The physician will determine the dosage based on the specific needs and therapeutic response of the child.

PRECAUTIONS AND WARNINGS
Take care not to contaminate the eyedropper when instilling the solution form of Neosporin. Do not let the dropper touch the eye.

POSSIBLE SIDE EFFECTS
Neosporin contains a combination of three antibiotics. Prolonged use of any antibiotic can cause the growth and multiplication of microorganisms that are unaffected by the drug. Such a "superinfection" may occur with the long-term use of Neosporin.

The most common side effect is an allergic reaction in children who are especially sensitive to the neomycin ingredient. Should this occur, consult the physician immediately.

Neo-Synephrine® 12 Hour Children's Nose Drops (OTC)

GENERIC NAME
Oxymetazoline hydrochloride (0.025 percent).

PRODUCT CATEGORY
Decongestant.

DOSAGE FORM
Liquid (for instillation in the nose).

WHY USED
It is used to reduce nasal congestion so that free breathing can be restored in children afflicted with the common cold, sinusitis, hay fever, or other allergies.

CHILDREN'S DOSAGE
Neo-Synephrine Children's Nose Drops are formulated for use in children between the ages of two and six years. It is not recommended for use in children under the age of two years. (Adult-strength Neo-Synephrine nose drops and nasal sprays are generally available for children over the age of six years.) The usual recommended dosage is to instill two or three drops instilled in each nostril twice a day, once in the morning and again in the evening.

PRECAUTIONS AND WARNINGS
Do not use this product for more than three days. If symptoms persist, consult a physician. The dispenser should not be used by more than one person, because of the risk of spreading an infection.

POSSIBLE SIDE EFFECTS
Side effects associated with the use of this product, which may include a burning or stinging sensation, sneezing, or an increase in nasal discharge, usually are the result of giving larger than recommended dosages.

Nilstat®

GENERIC NAME
Nystatin.

PRODUCT CATEGORY
Antifungal.

DOSAGE FORM
Oral suspension (cherry flavor).

WHY PRESCRIBED
It is used for the treatment of infections of the mouth caused by the yeast, *Candida albicans*, also known as "thrush."

CHILDREN'S DOSAGE
The physician will determine the exact dosage, which depends upon the age of the infant or child and the severity of the infection. The child should hold the oral suspension in the mouth as long as possible without swallowing.

PRECAUTIONS AND WARNINGS
This product should not be given to a child who is known to be hypersensitive (allergic) to ingredients of the preparation.

POSSIBLE SIDE EFFECTS
Among reported side effects are digestive disorders, including nausea, vomiting, and diarrhea.

Noctec®

GENERIC NAME
Chloral hydrate.

PRODUCT CATEGORY
Sedative/hypnotic (sleep-inducing drug).

DOSAGE FORM
Syrup and capsules.

WHY PRESCRIBED
It is used to help induce sleep and provide sedation.

CHILDREN'S DOSAGE
The usual dosage for children to induce sleep (hypnotic effect) is 50 milligrams per kilogram of body weight (1 kilogram = 2.2 pounds), given daily as a single dose or in two equally divided doses. The usual dosage to provide sedation is half this amount. In no case should a child receive more than 1 gram (1,000 milligrams) in a single dose. The capsules should be taken with liquid; the syrup may be taken in water, fruit juice, or ginger ale.

PRECAUTIONS AND WARNINGS
The prolonged use of Noctec, especially in excessive doses, can be habit forming. Sudden withdrawal of the drug after long-term use may result in delirium.

Do not give Noctec to children with kidney or liver disease or severe heart disease, unless the physician is aware of the medical history.

Noctec may lose its effectiveness as a sedative and sleep-inducing drug after continued administration for about two weeks.

POSSIBLE SIDE EFFECTS
The most common side effect is irritation of the stomach. Some children may also experience nausea, vomiting, diarrhea, unpleasant taste, drug-induced skin rashes, dizziness, and impaired coordination.

Overdosage with Noctec can result in coma.

Nostril® (OTC)

GENERIC NAME
Phenylephrine hydrochloride.

PRODUCT CATEGORY
Decongestant.

DOSAGE FORM
Liquid (to be sprayed into nostrils).

WHY USED
It is used to relieve nasal congestion (stuffy nose) in cases of the common cold, sinusitis, hay fever, and other respiratory allergies.

CHILDREN'S DOSAGE
The product is available in two strengths, 0.5 percent and 0.25 percent. The 0.5 percent formulation is intended for adults and children over the age of twelve years and should not be given to younger children except on the advice of a physician. The 0.25 percent formulation is recommended for children between the ages of six and twelve years. It should not be given to children under the age of six years without the advice of a physician. The usual recommended dosage for either type is one or two sprays into each nostril every four hours.

PRECAUTIONS AND WARNINGS
Do not exceed the recommended dosage and do not give the medication more frequently than once every four hours. Do not use the product for more than three days. If the symptoms persist, consult a physician.

POSSIBLE SIDE EFFECTS
Most reported side effects, including a burning or stinging sensation, sneezing, or increased nasal discharge, are the result of using larger than recommended dosages.

Nostrilla® (OTC)

GENERIC NAME
Oxymetazoline hydrochloride (0.05 percent).

PRODUCT CATEGORY
Decongestant.

DOSAGE FORM
Liquid (to be sprayed into the nostrils).

WHY USED
Nostrilla is used to provide prolonged (up to twelve hours) relief from the symptoms of nasal congestion (stuffy nose) associated with the common cold, sinusitis, hay fever, and other upper respiratory allergies.

CHILDREN'S DOSAGE
The usual recommended dosage for children over the age of six years is one or two sprays in each nostril twice a day, once in the morning and once in the evening.

PRECAUTIONS AND WARNINGS
This product should not be given to children under the age of six years without the advice and supervision of a physician. Do not use the product for more than three days. If the symptoms persist, consult a physician.

POSSIBLE SIDE EFFECTS
The most common side effects, which include a burning or stinging sensation, sneezing, or increased nasal discharge, are usually the result of using larger than recommended dosages.

Novafed®

GENERIC NAME
Pseudoephedrine hydrochloride.

PRODUCT CATEGORY
Decongestant.

DOSAGE FORM
Liquid and controlled-release capsules.

WHY PRESCRIBED
This product is used to relieve congestion in the nose or the eustachian tube that may be associated with the common cold, sinusitis, otitis media (middle ear inflammation), hay fever, or other upper respiratory allergies.

CHILDREN'S DOSAGE
The capsules are not recommended for children under the age of twelve years. For children over the age of twelve, the usual recommended dosage is one capsule every twelve hours. The liquid form of the product is available without a doctor's prescription. It should not be given to children under the age of two years without the advice and supervision of a physician. For older children, follow the directions on the label.

PRECAUTIONS AND WARNINGS
This product should not be given to children who are known to be hypersensitive to pseudoephedrine hydrochloride or to related drugs. It also should not be given to children with high blood pressure, diabetes, heart disease, or thyroid disease without a doctor's advice. The doctor should be advised of any other medications being taken by the child in order to prevent possible adverse effects of drug interactions.

POSSIBLE SIDE EFFECTS
Among reported side effects are rapid heartbeat (tachycardia), sensation of heartbeat (palpitations), headache, dizziness, nausea, tremors, insomnia, difficulty urinating, anxiety, restlessness, weakness, and breathing difficulty. Some side effects may vary with individual differences in sensitivity to the drug.

Novahistine® Elixir (OTC)

GENERIC NAME
This product contains in each teaspoonful (5 ml) phenylephrine hydrochloride (5 mg), chlorpheniramine maleate (2 mg), and alcohol (5 percent).

PRODUCT CATEGORY
Decongestant/antihistamine.

DOSAGE FORM
Elixir.

WHY USED
It is mainly used to relieve the symptoms of stuffy nose (nasal congestion) associated with allergies such as hay fever (allergic rhinitis). Novahistine is also used to unblock a congested Eustachian tube—the canal between the middle ear and the upper part of the throat that equalizes air pressure on either side of the eardrum.

CHILDREN'S DOSAGE

Age of Child	Teaspoonfuls (5 ml) Every Four Hours
Over 12 years	2
6–12 years	1
2–5 years	½

Do not give a child more than six doses during any 24-hour period. Do not give Novahistine to a child under the age of two years without medical advice.

PRECAUTIONS AND WARNINGS
Novahistine should be used with caution (if at all) in children with high blood pressure (hypertension), diabetes, heart disorders, or thyroid disease.

POSSIBLE SIDE EFFECTS
The most common side effects are drowsiness, nervousness, dizziness, and insomnia.

NTZ® Long Acting (OTC)

GENERIC NAME
Oxymetazoline hydrochloride (0.05 percent).

PRODUCT CATEGORY
Decongestant.

DOSAGE FORM
Nose drops and nasal spray.

WHY USED
It is used for prolonged (12 hours) relief from the symptoms of nasal congestion (stuffy nose) associated with the common cold, sinusitis, hay fever, or other upper respiratory allergies.

CHILDREN'S DOSAGE
The product is instilled in each nostril by spray or drops, according to the directions on the label, twice daily, once in the morning and again in the evening.

PRECAUTIONS AND WARNINGS
This product is not recommended for use in children under the age of six years. Do not use the product for more than three days. If the symptoms persist, consult a doctor. Use of the dispenser by more than one person may result in the spread of an infection.

POSSIBLE SIDE EFFECTS
The most common side effects, which include a burning or stinging sensation, sneezing, or increased nasal discharge, are usually the result of using excessive amounts of the medication.

Nucofed®

GENERIC NAME
This product contains in each capsule or 5 ml teaspoonful a combination of codeine phosphate (20 mg), pseudoephedrine hydrochloride (60 mg), and various other ingredients, including colorings and flavorings.

PRODUCT CATEGORY
Antitussive (cough suppressant)/decongestant.

DOSAGE FORM
Capsules and syrup.

WHY PRESCRIBED
This product is used to relieve the symptoms of coughing and congestion associated with the common cold, influenza, sinusitis, bronchitis, and other infections of the upper respiratory tract.

CHILDREN'S DOSAGE
The capsule form of this product is not recommended for children under the age of twelve years.

Age of Child	Teaspoonfuls (5 ml) of Syrup Every Six Hours
6–12 years	½
2–6 years	¼

This product should not be given to a child under the age of two years without the advice and supervision of a physician.

PRECAUTIONS AND WARNINGS
This product is not recommended for children whose coughing is associated with asthma, or emphysema, or when the cough is accompanied by excessive secretions. It also should not be given to a child affected by shortness of breath, high blood pressure, heart disease, diabetes, or thyroid disease, except with the advice and supervision of a physician. A child who is taking another medication should use Nucofed only with the advice and supervision of a physician. Codeine may be habit-forming.

POSSIBLE SIDE EFFECTS
Use of this product can cause or aggravate constipation. Excessive doses may result in nervousness, dizziness, or sleeplessness. The child also may experience difficulty urinating, headache, nausea and vomiting, drowsiness, changes in heartbeat, sweating, difficulty breathing, and loss of sensitivity to pain.

Nuprin® (OTC)

GENERIC NAME
Ibuprofen.

PRODUCT CATEGORY
Analgesic (pain reliever)/antipyretic (fever reducer)/anti-inflammatory (non-steroidal).

DOSAGE FORM
Tablets.

WHY USED
It is used for the relief of minor aches and pains that may be associated with the common cold, toothache, headache, backache, muscular aches, and arthritis pain. The product also may be used to reduce fever.

CHILDREN'S DOSAGE
This product should not be given to children under the age of twelve years without the advice and supervision of a physician. For children age twelve and older, the usual recommended dosage is one tablet every four to six hours, but not more than six tablets in any 24-hour period. The tablets can be taken with milk or food to reduce the possibility of mild heartburn or upset stomach experienced by some children taking the drug.

PRECAUTIONS AND WARNINGS
Ibuprofen should not be given to any child who is allergic to aspirin or related drugs, even though this product is aspirin-free. Do not give the product for more than three days if fever persists, or for more than ten days if pain continues or worsens or if new symptoms develop. The doctor should be advised about any other medication the child may be taking at the same time.

POSSIBLE SIDE EFFECTS
The most common side effects of ibuprofen use include nausea, abdominal pain, dizziness, and headache. Less frequently reported are constipation, diarrhea, swollen feet and legs, and tinnitus (ringing in the ears).

Orasone®

GENERIC NAME
Prednisone.

PRODUCT CATEGORY
Corticosteroid (synthetic glucocorticoid)/anti-inflammatory.

DOSAGE FORM
Tablets.

WHY PRESCRIBED
It is used in the treatment of a wide variety of inflammatory and allergic conditions. Orasone is often used in combination with other corticosteroids in treating disorders of the adrenal glands, to replace hormones normally produced by these glands.

CHILDREN'S DOSAGE
This depends on the type and severity of the condition being treated and the response of the child to Orasone therapy. The physician will individualize the dosage to the child's requirements.

PRECAUTIONS AND WARNINGS
Children should not be vaccinated against smallpox or be subjected to other immunization procedures while undergoing corticosteroid therapy. Because Orasone may interact with aspirin and many other prescription and nonprescription drugs, resulting in adverse effects, the doctor should be consulted about giving the child any additional medications while taking this product. Prednisone products may affect a child's response surgery, injury, or illness for up to two years after the drug has been discontinued. Thus, any doctor providing care for the child in the next two years should be advised of the child's previous use of the drug.

POSSIBLE SIDE EFFECTS
All drugs in the general class of corticosteroids, such as Orasone, are capable of causing a wide range of adverse effects. These are largely related to the dosage and the duration of therapy. Among the reported side effects are suppressed growth in children; accumulation of fatty deposits around the face, neck, or abdomen; nervousness; a decrease in bone tissue density (osteoporosis); increased susceptibility to infection; water retention, leading to swelling of the tissues (edema); euphoria; insomnia; skin changes; and increased susceptibility to bruising.

Ornade® Spansule® Capsules

GENERIC NAME
This product contains a combination of phenylpropanolamine hydrochloride (75 mg) and chlorpheniramine maleate (12 mg).

PRODUCT CATEGORY
Decongestant/antihistamine.

DOSAGE FORM
Capsules (sustained-release).

WHY PRESCRIBED
It is used to relieve the symptoms of runny nose, watery eyes, sneezing, itchy nose and throat, and nasal congestion that may be associated with the common cold or an upper respiratory tract allergy, such as hay fever.

CHILDREN'S DOSAGE
This product should not be used by children under the age of twelve years. For children twelve years of age and older, the usual recommended dose is one capsule every twelve hours.

PRECAUTIONS AND WARNINGS
This product should not be given to a child who is hypersensitive (allergic) to the ingredients, or to one with high blood pressure, diabetes, heart disease, or peptic ulcer. It should not be used to treat asthma or disorders of the lower respiratory tract. It should not be given to a child who is also taking other medications without first consulting a physician. The drugs may reduce mental alertness, increasing the risk of accidents, and may also cause excitability in children.

POSSIBLE SIDE EFFECTS
Use of larger than recommended dosages can increase the risk of side effects that include dry mouth, dilated pupils, muscle spasms, depressed breathing, excitability, depression, difficulty urinating, nausea and vomiting, blurred vision, and sensation of heartbeat (palpitations).

Otic Domeboro® Solution

GENERIC NAME
Acetic acid (2 percent) in aluminum acetate solution.

PRODUCT CATEGORY
Antibacterial/antifungal.

DOSAGE FORM
Liquid (for instillation directly into the outer ear canal).

WHY USED
It is used for the treatment of superficial infections of the external ear canal by microorganisms that are susceptible to the product.

CHILDREN'S DOSAGE
The usual dosage is four to six drops instilled into the outer ear canal every two to three hours.

PRECAUTIONS AND WARNINGS
This product is for external use only. It should not be allowed to come into contact with the eyes. If irritation or a hypersensitivity (allergic) reaction occurs, discontinue use of the product and consult a physician.

POSSIBLE SIDE EFFECTS
No serious side effects are expected from use of this product when used according to directions.

Otrivin® (OTC)

GENERIC NAME
Xylometazoline hydrochloride.

PRODUCT CATEGORY
Decongestant.

DOSAGE FORM
Nasal spray and nasal drops.

WHY USED
It is used to relieve the symptoms of nasal congestion (stuffy nose) associated with the common cold, sinusitis, and certain respiratory allergies, such as hay fever.

CHILDREN'S DOSAGE
This product is available without a doctor's prescription. Administer to children exactly as recommended on the label.

PRECAUTIONS AND WARNINGS
Do not use this product for more than three days. If symptoms persist, consult a physician. Use of the dispenser by more than one child may cause the spread of an infection.

POSSIBLE SIDE EFFECTS
Most side effects, which include a stinging or burning sensation, sneezing, or increased nasal discharge, are the result of using larger than recommended dosages.

Children's Panadol® (OTC)

GENERIC NAME
Acetaminophen.

PRODUCT CATEGORY
Analgesic (pain reliever)/antipyretic (fever reducer).

DOSAGE FORM
Chewable fruit-flavored tablets (80 mg), liquid (160 mg per 5 ml teaspoonful), drops (80 mg per 0.8 ml dropperful).

WHY USED
It is used to reduce fevers in children and to relieve the aches and pains associated with colds and influenza, earaches, headaches, teething, tonsillectomies, and vaccinations.

CHILDREN'S DOSAGE
The recommended dosage is based on the age and size of the child and generally ranges between 10 and 15 milligrams per kilogram of body weight (1 kilogram = 2.2 pounds). The drug may be given every four hours up to a maximum of five times in any 24-hour period.

Age of Child	Tablets Every Four Hours
2–3 years	2
4–5 years	3
6–8 years	4
9–10 years	5
11–12 years	6

For children under the age of two years, a physician should be consulted about the use of Children's Panadol Tablets. For dosages of Children's Panadol Liquid:

Age of Child	Teaspoonfuls (5 ml) Every 4 Hours
2–3 years	1
4–5 years	1½
6–8 years	2
9–10 years	2½
11–12 years	3

Children's Panadol® (OTC) (Continued)

For children under the age of two years, a physician should be consulted about the use of Children's Panadol Liquid. For dosages of Children's Panadol Drops:

Age of Child	Dropperfuls (0.8 ml) Every 4 Hours
2–3 years	2
4–5 years	3
6–8 years	4

For children under the age of two years, consult a physician about the use of Children's Panadol Drops.

PRECAUTIONS AND WARNINGS
Do not give Children's Panadol to a child who is under medical care without the knowledge and approval of a physician. The drug should not be continued for more than five days without physician supervision. The physician also should be consulted if symptoms persist or new symptoms develop while using acetaminophen products.

Unlike aspirin, acetaminophen has no ability to reduce redness and swelling (anti-inflammatory action).

POSSIBLE SIDE EFFECTS
Few side effects have been reported among children using acetaminophen products. An overdose of the product may result in liver disorders, marked by a yellowing of the skin and the whites of the eyes (jaundice) in some patients. If such effects are observed stop giving the drug and contact a physician or a poison control center immediately. A physician should also be consulted if there are signs of severe recurrent pain or high continued fever.

Panmycin®

GENERIC NAME
Tetracycline.

PRODUCT CATEGORY
Antibacterial/antiamebic/antirickettsial.

DOSAGE FORM
Capsules.

WHY PRESCRIBED
It is used to treat infections caused by a wide range of microorganisms, including contain species of bacteria, protozoa, and rickettsiae (intermediate in size between bacteria and viruses).

CHILDREN'S DOSAGE
This depends on the child's age and body weight. The usual total daily dosage of oral forms of tetracycline may range up to 25 to 50 milligrams per kilogram of body weight (1 kilogram = 2.2 pounds), given in equally divided doses. Tetracycline should not be given to children under the age of eight years, unless the physician determines that other antibiotics would be ineffective or inappropriate.

PRECAUTIONS AND WARNINGS
Tetracyclines may cause permanent discoloration of the teeth if given to children under the age of eight years.

Do not give the child antacids while he or she is being treated with tetracycline, since this could interfere with the effectiveness of the antibiotic.

Tetracycline should be used with caution (if at all) in children with impaired liver or kidney function.

POSSIBLE SIDE EFFECTS
The most common side effects include nausea, vomiting, diarrhea, heartburn, flatulence (gas), and loss of appetite (anorexia). Tetracycline is capable of causing potentially more serious side effects in some patients, including damage to the blood-forming tissues and a severe generalized allergic reaction (anaphylactic shock).

Some children taking tetracycline may experience severe skin eruptions and rashes when exposed to strong sunlight. These exaggerated "sunburn reactions" usually disappear days or weeks after therapy with tetracycline has been discontinued.

Paraflex®

GENERIC NAME
Chlorzoxazone (250 mg).

PRODUCT CATEGORY
Skeletal muscle relaxant.

DOSAGE FORM
Tablets.

WHY PRESCRIBED
It is used to help relieve the symptoms of painful muscle spasms.

CHILDREN'S DOSAGE
This depends on the severity of symptoms and the child's response to Paraflex therapy. The usual dosage is one-half to two tablets (125 mg to 500 mg), depending on the child's age and body weight, given three or four times daily.

PRECAUTIONS AND WARNINGS
Paraflex should be used with caution in children with known allergies, especially allergic reactions to drugs. Use of Paraflex should be discontinued at the first sign of a skin rash or redness and itching. Consult the physician at once if such a reaction occurs.

POSSIBLE SIDE EFFECTS
Paraflex rarely causes significant side effects. Some children may experience drowsiness, lightheadedness, a general feeling of being unwell (malaise), or overstimulation.

paregoric (generic)

BRAND NAMES
This drug is not marketed under a brand name. An alternative generic name is camphorated tincture of opium.

PRODUCT CATEGORY
Antidiarrheal.

DOSAGE FORM
Liquid.

WHY PRESCRIBED
It is used in the treatment of diarrhea. The drug acts by slowing down the movements (peristalsis) of the intestines.

CHILDREN'S DOSAGE
This depends on the weight of the child. The usual dosage is 0.25 to 0.5 milliliters per kilogram of body weight (1 kilogram = 2.2 pounds), given one to four times a day.

PRECAUTIONS AND WARNINGS
Paregoric should not be used to treat diarrhea caused by poisons or infectious agents until the material has been eliminated from the digestive tract. Prolonged use of the drug may lead to physical dependence on paregoric. This product should NOT be confused with *opium tincture*, which is twenty-five times more potent.

POSSIBLE SIDE EFFECTS
Some children may experience nausea or vomiting, dizziness, lightheadedness, sedation, euphoria or other behavioral changes, depressed breathing, itching, or constipation.

Pathocil®

GENERIC NAME
Dicloxacillin sodium monohydrate.

PRODUCT CATEGORY
Antibiotic (semisynthetic penicillin).

DOSAGE FORM
Capsules and oral suspension.

WHY PRESCRIBED
It is used in the treatment of certain skin and respiratory tract infections that are caused by bacteria susceptible to dicloxacillin, particularly strains of microorganisms that do not respond to penicillin or that are capable of destroying penicillin.

CHILDREN'S DOSAGE
This depends largely on the severity of the infection and the child's age and weight. The usual daily dosages range from 12.5 to 25 milligrams per kilogram of body weight (1 kilogram = 2.2 pounds), given in equally divided doses every six hours. The drug should be given one to two hours before a meal, because it is best absorbed on an empty stomach.

PRECAUTIONS AND WARNINGS
This product should not be given to a child who has shown a hypersensitivity (allergy) to penicillin or other similar antibiotics. If symptoms of an allergic reaction are noted, use of the drug should be discontinued and a physician should be notified immediately. Oral forms of antibiotics should be used with caution in children with symptoms of digestive system upsets, including diarrhea, nausea, and vomiting.

POSSIBLE SIDE EFFECTS
Among reported side effects are gastrointestinal disorders, including nausea, vomiting, flatulence (gas), and loose stools, as well as skin rashes, urticaria (hives), and itching.

Pedialyte®

GENERIC NAME
This product contains a combination of water, dextrose, potassium citrate, sodium chloride, and sodium citrate.

PRODUCT CATEGORY
Electrolyte replacement.

DOSAGE FORM
Liquid (fruit flavor).

WHY PRESCRIBED
It is given to infants and children with mild to moderate diarrhea, and to those recovering from severe diarrhea, to help restore fluid and electrolyte balance.

CHILDREN'S DOSAGE
The exact dosage varies according to the age and weight of the child ranging and the degree of dehydration. The physician will individualize the dosage.

PRECAUTIONS AND WARNINGS
The total daily intake should be adjusted according to the needs and response of the child.

POSSIBLE SIDE EFFECTS
No serious side effects are expected.

Pediamycin®

GENERIC NAME
Erythromycin ethylsuccinate.

PRODUCT CATEGORY
Antibiotic.

DOSAGE FORM
Oral suspension.

WHY PRESCRIBED
Pediamycin, as well as other forms of erythromycin, is used to treat mild to moderate bacterial infections, especially when the child is known to be allergic to penicillin or when the bacteria do not respond to penicillin.

CHILDREN'S DOSAGE
This depends largely on the severity of the infection and the child's age and weight. The usual total daily dosage is 30 to 50 milligrams per kilogram of body weight (1 kilogram = 2.2 pounds), given in divided doses two to four times per day. In treating particularly severe infections, the physician may double this amount.

PRECAUTIONS AND WARNINGS
Children should take Pediamycin at the times and in the exact amounts prescribed by the physician. Taking more than the prescribed amount is not only wasteful but can cause stomach discomfort, nausea, vomiting, and diarrhea.

Long-term use of any antibiotic may result in the development of a "superinfection"—the growth and multiplication in the body of fungi and other microorganisms that are unaffected by the drug. Dispose of any remaining suspension or drops once the course of therapy has been successfully completed.

POSSIBLE SIDE EFFECTS
Pediamycin, like other forms of erythromycin, is a relatively safe antibiotic, and serious side effects are uncommon. Most common adverse effects are gastrointestinal upsets, such as nausea, vomiting, diarrhea, and stomach cramps. Allergic reactions may include urticaria (hives) and skin rashes.

Pediazole®

GENERIC NAME
This product contains a combination of erythromycin ethylsuccinate and sulfisoxazole acetyl.

PRODUCT CATEGORY
Antibiotic.

DOSAGE FORM
Liquid (oral suspension).

WHY PRESCRIBED
It is used to treat children with infections of the middle ear (acute otitis media) caused by a specific type of bacteria (*Hemophilus influenzae*).

CHILDREN'S DOSAGE
This depends on the weight of the child. For example, the usual dosage for children who weight 8 kilograms (18 pounds) is one-half teaspoonful (2.5 ml) every six hours; for those who weigh 16 kilograms (35 pounds), one teaspoonful every six hours; and for those who weigh over 45 kilograms (100 pounds), two teaspoonfuls every six hours. Pediazole should not be given to children under the age of two months.

PRECAUTIONS AND WARNINGS
Pediazole should not be given to children with a known hypersensitivity (allergy) to either erythromycin or the sulfonamides (sulfa drugs).

Pediazole should be given with caution (if at all) to children with a disease of the kidneys or liver, severe allergies, or bronchial asthma.

Be sure the child drinks plenty of water or other fluids while taking Pediazole. This helps prevent the formation of crystals of the sulfa drug ingredient, which could damage the kidneys.

POSSIBLE SIDE EFFECTS
The most commonly reported side effects are abdominal pain or discomfort, nausea, vomiting, dizziness, and headache. Some patients taking this class of fixed-combination drug may experience allergic or hypersensitivity reactions ranging from skin rashes to life-threatening anaphylactic shock.

Stop giving Pediazole to a child who develops a skin rash, a sudden sore throat, or yellowness of the skin (jaundice), and consult a physician immediately.

penicillin G (generic)

BRAND NAMES
Bicillin®, Pentids®, Pfizerpen G®, SK-Penicillin G®.

PRODUCT CATEGORY
Broad-spectrum antibiotic.

DOSAGE FORM
Tablets and oral solution (as potassium salt); also available as benzathine derivative (Bicillin® tablets).

WHY PRESCRIBED
It is used to treat a wide variety of bacterial infections. (Penicillin has no effect against fungal or viral infections.)

CHILDREN'S DOSAGE
This depends on the severity of the infection, the type of bacteria involved, and the age and weight of the child. For example, the usual total daily dosage for infants and small children is 15 to 56 milligrams (25,000 to 90,000 units) per kilogram of body weight (1 kilogram = 2.2 pounds), given in three to six divided doses. To obtain the maximum therapeutic benefit, penicillin G should be given on an empty stomach either thirty minutes before or two hours after a meal. Otherwise, stomach acids can impair the effectiveness of the antibiotic.

PRECAUTIONS AND WARNINGS
Penicillin should never be given to a child with a known allergy to it. Such hypersensitivity to the drug is greater in children who have experienced other allergies such as hay fever or hives (urticaria) or who have asthma.

Long-term use of any antibiotic may result in the development of a "superinfection"—the growth and multiplication in the body of fungi and other microorganisms that are not affected by the drug. Dispose of any remaining tablets or solution of penicillin once the course of therapy has been successfully completed.

POSSIBLE SIDE EFFECTS
The most commonly reported side effects are upset stomach, abdominal discomfort or pain, diarrhea, a black "hairy" tongue, and drug-induced fever. In children who are allergic to the antibiotic, penicillin can cause a severe and potentially fatal reaction (anaphylactic shock).

penicillin VK (generic)

BRAND NAMES
Betapen VK®, Ledercillin VK®, Pen-Vee K®, Robicillin VK®, SK-Penicillin VK®, V-Cillin K®, Veetids®.

PRODUCT CATEGORY
Broad-spectrum/antibiotic.

DOSAGE FORM
Tablets and oral solution.

WHY PRESCRIBED
It is used to treat a wide variety of bacterial infections. (Penicillin has no effect against fungal or viral infections).

CHILDREN'S DOSAGE
This depends on the severity of the infection, the type of bacteria involved, and the age and weight of the child. For example, the usual total daily dosage for infants and small children is 25,000 to 90,000 units (15 to 56 milligrams) per kilogram of body weight (1 kilogram = 2.2 pounds), given in three to six divided doses. Penicillin VK is not as easily affected by stomach acid as penicillin G. Thus, it is not necessary to take it on an empty stomach.

PRECAUTIONS AND WARNINGS
Penicillin should never be given to a child with a known allergy to it. Such hypersensitivity to the drug is greater in children who have experienced other allergies such as hay fever or hives (urticaria) or who have asthma.

Long-term use of any antibiotic may result in the development of a "superinfection"—the growth and multiplication in the body of fungi and other microorganisms that are not affected by the drug. Dispose of any remaining tablets or oral solution of penicillin once the course of therapy has been successfully completed.

POSSIBLE SIDE EFFECTS
The most commonly reported side effects are upset stomach, abdominal discomfort or pain, diarrhea, a black "hairy" tongue, and drug-induced fever. In children who are hypersensitive to the antibiotic, penicillin can cause a severe and potentially fatal allergic reaction (anaphylactic shock).

Pentids®

GENERIC NAME
Penicillin G.

PRODUCT CATEGORY
Broad-spectrum antibiotic.

DOSAGE FORM
Tablets and oral solution.

WHY PRESCRIBED
It is used to treat a wide variety of mild to moderately severe bacterial infections.

CHILDREN'S DOSAGE
This depends on the severity of the infection, the type of bacteria involved, and the age and weight of the child. For example, the usual total daily dosage for infants and small children is 15 to 56 milligrams (25,000 to 90,000 units) per kilogram of body weight (1 kilogram = 2.2 pounds), given in three to six divided doses. To obtain the maximum therapeutic benefit, Pentids should be given on an empty stomach either thirty minutes before or at least two hours after a meal. Otherwise, natural stomach acids can impair the effectiveness of the antibiotic.

PRECAUTIONS AND WARNINGS
Penicillin should never be given to a child with a known allergy to it. Such hypersensitivity to the drug is greater in children who have experienced other allergies such as hay fever or hives (urticaria) or who have asthma.

Long-term use of any antibiotic may result in the development of a "superinfection"—the growth and multiplication in the body of fungi and other microorganisms that are unaffected by the drug. Dispose of any remaining tablets or oral solution once the course of therapy has been successfully completed.

POSSIBLE SIDE EFFECTS
The most commonly reported side effects are upset stomach, abdominal discomfort or pain, diarrhea, a black "hairy" tongue, and drug-induced fever. In children who are allergic to the antibiotic, penicillin can cause a severe and potentially fatal reaction (anaphylactic shock).

Pen-Vee K®

GENERIC NAME
Penicillin VK.

PRODUCT CATEGORY
Broad-spectrum/antibiotic.

DOSAGE FORM
Tablets and oral solution.

WHY PRESCRIBED
It is used to treat a wide variety of bacterial infections.

CHILDREN'S DOSAGE
This depends on the severity of the infection, the type of bacteria involved, and the age and weight of the child. For example, the usual total daily dosage for infants and small children is 25,000 to 90,000 units (15 to 56 milligrams) per kilogram of body weight (1 kilogram = 2.2 pounds), given in three to six divided doses. Penicillin VK products are not as easily affected by stomach acids as the penicillin G forms of the antibiotic. Thus, it is not necessary to take the drug on an empty stomach.

PRECAUTIONS AND WARNINGS
Penicillin should never be given to a child with a known allergy to it. Such hypersensitivity to the drug is greater in children who have experienced other allergies such as hay fever or hives (urticaria) or who have asthma.

Long-term use of any antibiotic may result in the development of a "superinfection"—the growth and multiplication of fungi and other microorganisms that are not affected by the drug. Dispose of any remaining tablets or oral solution once the course of therapy has been successfully completed.

POSSIBLE SIDE EFFECTS
The most commonly reported side effects are upset stomach, abdominal discomfort or pain, diarrhea, a black "hairy" tongue, and drug-induced fever. In children who are hypersensitive to the antibiotic, penicillin can cause a severe and potentially fatal allergic reaction (anaphylactic shock).

Pepto-Bismol® (OTC)

GENERIC NAME
Bismuth subsalicylate.

PRODUCT CATEGORY
Antidiarrheal.

DOSAGE FORM
Liquid (oral suspension) and chewable tablets.

WHY USED
It is used mainly to control common diarrhea and may also be useful for the relief of upset stomach, indigestion, nausea, and heartburn.

CHILDREN'S DOSAGE
Pepto-Bismol is available without a doctor's prescription. Administer to children exactly as the label recommends.

PRECAUTIONS AND WARNINGS
This product contains salicylates, which are chemically related to aspirin. When taken with aspirin, tinnitus (ringing in the ears) may occur, requiring that use of the product be discontinued. It should not be given to a child with a known allergy to aspirin. The product should not be given to children, including teenagers, during or after recovery from chickenpox or influenza without first consulting the doctor. A doctor also should be consulted if the child is taking medication for diabetes or certain other chronic disorders. If the child's diarrhea continues for more than two days or is accompanied by a high fever, discontinue use of the product and consult a physician.

POSSIBLE SIDE EFFECTS
Pepto-Bismol may cause a harmless and temporary darkening of the tongue and stools in some children. The bismuth ingredient also may result in the impaction of feces in some infants taking this product.

Periactin®

GENERIC NAME
Cyproheptadine hydrochloride.

PRODUCT FORM
Antihistamine/antiserotoneric.

DOSAGE FORM
Syrup and tablets.

WHY PRESCRIBED
It is used mainly to relieve the symptoms of hay fever (allergic rhinitis), allergic conjunctivitis, and allergic inflammations of the skin.

CHILDREN'S DOSAGE
This depends largely on the age and weight or body surface area of the child. The usual total daily dosage for children is 0.25 milligrams per kilogram of body weight (1 kilogram = 2.2 pounds), given in divided doses two or three times a day. The manufacturer recommends that the physician adjust the dosage according to the individual needs and response of the child.

PRECAUTIONS AND WARNINGS
An overdose of Periactin in infants and children can cause hallucinations, convulsions, and even death.

The drug should be used with caution (if at all) in children with bronchial asthma, heart disease, thyroid disease, or high blood pressure (hypertension).

POSSIBLE SIDE EFFECTS
The most commonly reported side effects include sedation; thickening of the secretions in the lower air passages; dryness of the mouth, nose, and throat; impaired coordination; and abdominal discomfort.

Phenergan® Syrup

GENERIC NAME
Promethazine hydrochloride.

PRODUCT CATEGORY
Antihistamine.

DOSAGE FORM
Syrup, tablets and suppositories.

WHY PRESCRIBED
It is used to prevent or relieve the symptoms of various allergies, such as hay fever (allergic rhinitis). In addition, Phenergan may be used as a sedative in children and to prevent motion sickness, nausea, vomiting, and dizziness.

CHILDREN'S DOSAGE
This depends largely on the specific use for which the drug is prescribed as well as the individual needs and response of the child. For example, the usual dosage in the treatment of allergies is a single 25 milligram dose at bedtime at the start of therapy. Thereafter, the smallest amount of the drug that will maintain relief from symptoms is given.

PRECAUTIONS AND WARNINGS
Do not give Phenergan to a child with a known sensitivity to the drug. The drug should not be given to a child under the age of two years without the advice of a physician. It should be used with caution in a child with epilepsy.

POSSIBLE SIDE EFFECTS
The most common side effect is drowsiness (which also is a therapeutic effect when the drug is used as a sedative). Other adverse effects may include blurred vision, dry mouth, dizziness, increased or lowered blood pressure, skin rash, and nausea and vomiting.

phenobarbital (generic)

BRAND NAMES
Solfoton®.

PRODUCT CATEGORY
Sedative/anticonvulsant (barbiturate).

DOSAGE FORM
Tablets, capsules, and elixir.

WHY PRESCRIBED
It is used to calm anxiety and help induce sleep (sedative action) and, alone or in combination with other drugs, to prevent or control convulsive seizures (anticonvulsant or antiepileptic action).

CHILDREN'S DOSAGE
This depends on the condition being treated and the body weight of the child. For example, a dosage to control convulsions may be 15 to 50 milligrams two to three times daily. For sedation of children, the total daily dosage may be 6 milligrams per kilogram of body weight, given in divided doses three times a day. (When timed-release forms of phenobarbital are prescribed, the dosage schedule will be less frequent.) The timed-release form is not recommended for children less than twelve years of age.

PRECAUTIONS AND WARNINGS
Children with an inborn (heredity) error of metabolism known as porphyria must not take phenobarbital or other barbiturates. The drug should be used with caution (if at all) in children with a disease of the kidneys or liver.

POSSIBLE SIDE EFFECTS
The most commonly reported side effects are drowsiness (which is a therapeutic effect when phenobarbital is taken as a sedative), dizziness, depression, vomiting, diarrhea, impaired breathing, and allergic reactions such as skin rashes.

Overdosage with phenobarbital can be fatal.

Polycillin®

GENERIC NAME
Ampicillin.

PRODUCT CATEGORY
Broad-spectrum antibiotic (semisynthetic penicillin).

DOSAGE FORM
Capsules and oral suspension.

WHY PRESCRIBED
This product is used to treat a wide range of bacterial infections in children, including those that involve the middle ear (otitis media), stomach and intestines (gastrointestinal tract), urinary tract, respiratory tract, the membranes that cover the brain (meningitis), and the skin.

CHILDREN'S DOSAGE
This depends largely on the severity of the infection and the age and body weight of the child. The site of the infection can also affect the dosage. For example, the usual dosage for children with an infection of the respiratory tract is 250 milligrams every six hours. However, if the child weighs less than 20 kilograms (44 pounds), the total daily dosage is 50 milligrams per kilogram of body weight (1 kilogram = 2.2 pounds), given in equally divided doses at intervals of six or eight hours. If it is kept refrigerated, ampicillin suspension remains stable for two weeks.

PRECAUTIONS AND WARNINGS
Polycillin should never be given to a child with a known allergic reaction to it or to penicillin. Adverse reactions are more likely if the child has experienced other allergies, such as hay fever or hives (urticaria).

POSSIBLE SIDE EFFECTS
The most common side effects are diarrhea and skin rashes. Some children may also experience nausea and vomiting. More serious side effects are relatively uncommon.

Polymox®

GENERIC NAME
Amoxicillin.

PRODUCT CATEGORY
Broad-spectrum antibiotic (semisynthetic penicillin).

DOSAGE FORM
Capsules oral suspension.

WHY PRESCRIBED
Polymox is used to treat a wide range of bacterial infections in children, including those that involve the ear, nose, and throat, urinary tract, skin, and lower part of the respiratory tract (air passages leading to the lungs).

CHILDREN'S DOSAGE
This depends largely on the severity of the infection and the child's age and weight. The usual total daily dosage is 20 milligrams per kilogram of body weight (1 kilogram = 2.2 pounds), given in divided doses every eight hours. For severe infections, the doctor may double the size of the dose. Be sure to shake the bottle well before giving the oral suspension.

PRECAUTIONS AND WARNINGS
Polymox should never be given to a child with a known allergic reaction to it or to penicillin. Adverse reactions are more likely if the child has experienced other allergies, such as asthma, hay fever, or hives (urticaria).

Long-term use of any antibiotic may result in the development of a "superinfection"—an overgrowth in the body of fungi and other microorganisms that are not affected by the drug. Dispose of any remaining Polymox once the course of therapy has been successfully completed.

POSSIBLE SIDE EFFECTS
Some children taking Polymox may experience diarrhea, nausea, vomiting, or skin rashes. More serious side effects are relatively uncommon.

Poly-Vi-Flor®

GENERIC NAME
This product contains (in drops) a combination of vitamins A, B6, B12, C, D, E, niacin, riboflavin, thiamine, and fluoride. The tablets contain, in addition, folic acid, copper, iron, and zinc. Drops and tablets contain iron, if so labeled.

PRODUCT CATEGORY
Multivitamin supplement with minerals and fluoride.

DOSAGE FORM
Infants' drops and chewable tablets.

WHY PRESCRIBED
It is used in children to correct vitamin deficiencies and to prevent or minimize the development of caries (dental cavities).

CHILDREN'S DOSAGE
This depends on the child's needs for vitamin supplements and the fluoride content of the local drinking water. The physician will determine the best dosage to meet individual requirements.

PRECAUTIONS AND WARNINGS
An excessive amount of fluoride can be harmful, especially if the drinking water contains fluoride in excess of 0.7 ppm (parts per million). Do not give the child more Poly-Vi-Flor than is prescribed by the physician.

POSSIBLE SIDE EFFECTS
Large amounts of fluoride can damage the teeth. Some children may also experience an allergic rash, upset stomach, weakness, itching (pruritus), and headache.

The overuse of certain vitamins, particularly vitamins A and D, can result in an accumulation of them in the body and potentially toxic (poisonous) effects.

Povan®

GENERIC NAME
Pyrvinium pamoate.

PRODUCT CATEGORY
Anthelmintic (antiparasitic).

DOSAGE FORM
Filmseal® (film-coated) tablets.

WHY PRESCRIBED
It is used in the treatment of pinworm infections (enterobiasis).

CHILDREN'S DOSAGE
This depends on the weight of the child. The usual total dosage is 5 milligrams per kilogram of body weight (1 pound = 2.2 pounds), administered as a single dose only once. If required, this dose may be repeated in two or three weeks.

PRECAUTIONS AND WARNINGS
Pyrvinium pamoate is a red dye. Unless the tablets are swallowed whole, they can stain the child's teeth. Also, the child's stools may be stained a bright red. If the child vomits, the vomit may also be stained red. Although this dye will stain most materials, it is harmless to the child.

POSSIBLE SIDE EFFECTS
Vomiting is a relatively common side effect. Other side effects may include diarrhea, nausea, cramps, and various allergic reactions. The gastrointestinal side effects are more frequent in older children who receive larger doses because of their greater body weight.

Primatene® Mist and Mist Suspension (OTC)

GENERIC NAME
Epinephrine (0.5 percent) in mist; as bitartrate (0.5 percent) in mist suspension.

PRODUCT CATEGORY
Bronchodilator/antiasthmatic.

DOSAGE FORM
Aerosol.

WHY USED
It helps relieve wheezing and shortness of breath in children with bronchial asthma.

CHILDREN'S DOSAGE
Primatene Mist is available without a doctor's prescription. If prompt relief is not obtained after following directions on the label (usually one or two applications), consult a physician.

PRECAUTIONS AND WARNINGS
Do not give a child Primatene Mist unless a medical diagnosis of asthma has been made. Overuse of aerosol bronchodilatos can be dangerous. Medical supervision of asthma, especially in children, is extremely important.

POSSIBLE SIDE EFFECTS
Serious side effects are uncommon. However, overdependence on treatment that is not effective may permit the condition to progress to a point where it becomes a direct threat to life.

If the child's symptoms fail to diminish, consult a doctor.

Primatene® Tablets (OTC)

GENERIC NAME
This product is sold in two formulations, depending on state prescription regulations. The "M" formula, available in states where a prescription is required for phenobarbital products, contains ephedrine hydrochloride (24 mg), theophylline (119 mg), and pyrilamine maleate (16.6 mg). In other states, a "P" formula product is available, containing phenobarbital (8 mg) instead of pyrilamine maleate.

PRODUCT CATEGORY
Bronchodilator/antiasthmatic.

DOSAGE FORM
Tablets.

WHY USED
It helps relieve wheezing and shortness of breath in children with bronchial asthma.

CHILDREN'S DOSAGE
Primatene Tablets are generally available without a doctor's prescription in the "M" formulation, while "P" formula Primatene Tablets may require a doctor's prescription. Use either product exactly as the label recommends. A doctor should be consulted about the use of Primatene Tablets for children under six years of age.

PRECAUTIONS AND WARNINGS
Do not give Primatene Tablets to a child unless a medical diagnosis of asthma has been made. Do not give this product to children with heart disease, high blood pressure (hypertension), or diabetes unless approved by a physician.

Children with symptoms of asthma should be examined by a physician. The most effective treatment often involves the administration of more potent prescription drugs.

If the child's symptoms fail to diminish, seek medical attention at once.

POSSIBLE SIDE EFFECTS
Some children may experience nervousness, restlessness, and sleeplessness. Should any of these side effects occur, stop giving the child Primatene Tablets and consult a doctor.

The pyrilamine maleate ingredient in the "M" formula may cause drowsiness. Excessive amounts of the antihistamine can cause potentially serious side effects. The phenobarbital in the "P" formula can be habit-forming.

Principen®

GENERIC NAME
Ampicillin.

PRODUCT CATEGORY
Broad-spectrum antibiotic (semisynthetic penicillin).

DOSAGE FORM
Capsules and oral suspension.

WHY PRESCRIBED
Principen is used to treat a wide range of bacterial infections in children, including those that involve the respiratory tract, the stomach and intestines (gastrointestinal tract), and the urinary tract.

CHILDREN'S DOSAGE
This depends largely on the type and severity of the infection and the child's age and weight. For children weighing less than 20 kilograms (44 pounds), the usual total daily dose for a respiratory tract infection is 50 milligrams per kilogram of body weight (1 kilogram = 2.2 pounds), given in three or four equally divided doses. For an infection of the urinary or the gastrointestinal tract, the total daily dosage may be 100 milligrams per kilogram of body weight, given in four equally divided doses.

PRECAUTIONS AND WARNINGS
This product should not be given to a child with a known allergic reaction to it or to pencillin. Adverse reactions are more likely if the child has experienced other allergies such as hay fever or hives (urticaria) or has asthma.

POSSIBLE SIDE EFFECTS
The most common side effects are diarrhea and skin rashes. Some children may also experience nausea and vomiting. More serious side effects are relatively uncommon.

Proventil®

GENERIC NAME
Albuterol sulfate.

PRODUCT CATEGORY
Bronchodilator.

DOSAGE FORM
Syrup, tablets, aerosol.

WHY PRESCRIBED
Proventil is used to prevent and relieve the symptoms of bronchospasms in children with bronchial asthma or other forms of disease causing obstruction of the air passages to the lungs.

CHILDREN'S DOSAGE
The tablet and aerosol forms of the drug are not recommended for children under the age of twelve years. The syrup form of Proventil is not recommended for children under the age of two years. The usual starting dose for children between the ages of two and six years is based on body weight and should not exceed one teaspoonful of syrup three times a day; for children between six and fourteen, the initial dosage may be one teaspoonful up to four times a day. The usual starting dose in tablet form, for children over the age of twelve years, is 2 to 4 milligrams three to four times a day. The physician may adjust the dosage later according to the needs and response of the child.

PRECAUTIONS AND WARNINGS
Albuterol should not be given to any child who is known to be hypersensitive (allergic) to the drug. It should be used with caution (if at all) in children with heart disease, high blood pressure, or thyroid disease. Large doses may aggravate diabetes. Excessive doses also can lead to severe asthmatic reactions that may be fatal.

POSSIBLE SIDE EFFECTS
The most commonly reported side effects include nervousness, headache, tremors, dizziness, insomnia, sensation of heartbeat (palpitations), rapid heartbeat (tachycardia), nausea, irritability, and muscle cramps.

Pyridium®

GENERIC NAME
Phenazopyridine hydrochloride.

PRODUCT CATEGORY
Analgesic (urinary tract).

DOSAGE FORM
Tablets.

WHY PRESCRIBED
It is used to relieve the symptoms of pain and burning of the bladder and urethra caused by infection or irritation of the lower part of the urinary tract.

CHILDREN'S DOSAGE
The physician will determine the most appropriate dosage based on the age and weight of the child and the severity of the symptoms.

PRECAUTIONS AND WARNINGS
Administer Pyridium to a child exactly as prescribed. An excessive amount can cause toxic (poisonous) reactions.

Pyridium should not be given to a child with impaired kidney function. Discontinue the use of this drug and consult the physician at the first sign of jaundice (yellowness of the skin or whites of the eyes).

POSSIBLE SIDE EFFECTS
The most commonly reported side effect is upset stomach or other disturbances of the gastrointestinal tract. Overdosage may cause damage to the kidneys or liver.

The use of Pyridium may cause the urine to turn red or orange. Be sure to tell the child that this is absolutely harmless and will disappear once the course of therapy has been successfully completed. Large doses also may result in changes in skin coloring.

Quibron®

GENERIC NAME
This product contains in each capsule or tablespoonful (15 ml) a combination of theophylline (150 mg) and guaifenesin (90 mg).

PRODUCT CATEGORY
Bronchodilator/antiasthmatic/expectorant.

DOSAGE FORM
Soft gelatin capsules and liquid.

WHY PRESCRIBED
It is used to relieve wheezing and shortness of breath in children with bronchial asthma. It also helps loosen phlegm and mucus in the air passages.

CHILDREN'S DOSAGE
This depends on the child's age and weight and the severity of the symptoms. The physician will adjust the dosage to the needs of the individual child.

PRECAUTIONS AND WARNINGS
Do not give the child any other drugs at the same time as Quibron without the knowledge and advice of the physician. This product should be used with caution in children with heart disease, high blood pressure (hypertension), or thyroid disease.

POSSIBLE SIDE EFFECTS
Most side effects are related to the use of excessive amounts of the drug. These include nervousness, nausea, vomiting, abdominal pain, headache, diarrhea, restlessness, irritability, muscle twitching, flushing, low blood pressure (hypotension), rapid heartbeat (tachycardia), sensation of heartbeat (palpitations), and excitability. In most cases, the frequency and severity of these side effects can be controlled when the physician adjusts the dosage.

Respbid®

GENERIC NAME
Theophylline.

PRODUCT CATEGORY
Bronchodilator.

DOSAGE FORM
Tablets (timed-release).

WHY PRESCRIBED
It is used to prevent and relieve the symptoms of asthma and reversible bronchospasm associated with chronic bronchitis.

CHILDREN'S DOSAGE
Respbid is not recommended for use in children under the age of six years. Because of variations in individual responses to theophylline and differences in body weights of children, the physician will individualize the dosage, with occasional adjustments to larger or smaller amounts according to the needs and reactions of the child to the drug.

PRECAUTIONS AND WARNINGS
Respbid tablets should not be given to a child who has a known hypersensitivity (allergy) to the drug. Reactions of small children should be observed closely as they may not complain of sensations such as rapid heartbeat or other changes in heart rhythms that can indicate an intolerance to the drug. Caution should be exercised in giving the child caffeine beverages, such as colas, or large amountb of chocolate, which can increase the effects of theophylline. If the child is taking any other medications, particularly drugs for respiratory disorders, the doctor should be consulted. Do not give the child doses that are larger than prescribed or for a longer period of time than recommended unless advised by a doctor.

POSSIBLE SIDE EFFECTS
Most adverse effects are related to excessive doses of the drug. Common side effects involve the digestive tract, including nausea, vomiting, abdominal pain, loss of appetite, and stomach irritation leading to bloody vomit, or central nervous system reactions, such as headache, irritability, dizziness, restlessness, nervousness, and convulsions.

Retet®

GENERIC NAME
Tetracycline.

PRODUCT CATEGORY
Antibacterial/antiamebic/antirickettsial.

DOSAGE FORM
Capsules.

WHY PRESCRIBED
It is used to treat infections caused by a wide range of microorganisms, including certain species of bacteria, protozoa, and rickettsiae (intermediate in size between bacteria and viruses).

CHILDREN'S DOSAGE
This depends on the child's age and weight. The usual total daily dosage of tetracyclines (to be taken by mouth) is 25 to 50 milligrams per kilogram of body weight (1 kilogram = 2.2 pounds), given in two to four equally divided doses. Tetracycline should not be given to children under the age of eight, unless the physician determines that other antibiotics would be ineffective or inappropriate.

PRECAUTIONS AND WARNINGS
Tetracycline may cause permanent discoloration of the teeth if given to children under the age of eight.

Do not give the child antacids while he or she is being treated with tetracycline, since this could interfere with the effectiveness of the antibiotic.

Tetracycline should be used with caution (if at all) in children with impaired function of the liver or kidneys.

POSSIBLE SIDE EFFECTS
The most common side effects include nausea, vomiting, diarrhea, heartburn, flatulence (gas), and loss of appetite (anorexia). Tetracycline is capable of causing potentially more serious side effects in some patients, including damage to the blood-forming tissues and a severe generalized allergic reaction (anaphylactic shock).

Some children (as well as adults) taking tetracycline may experience severe skin eruptions and rashes when exposed to strong sunlight. These exaggerated "sunburn reactions" usually disappear days or weeks after therapy with tetracycline has been discontinued.

Rheaban® (OTC)

GENERIC NAME
Activated attapulgite.

PRODUCT CATEGORY
Antidiarrheal.

DOSAGE FORM
Liquid (oral suspension) and tablets.

WHY USED
It is used to control common diarrhea.

CHILDREN'S DOSAGE
Rheaban is available without a doctor's prescription. Administer to children exactly as the label recommends.

PRECAUTIONS AND WARNINGS
Rheaban should not be given to children under the age of three years unless directed by a physician. If the child's diarrhea continues for more than two days, or is accompanied by a high fever, consult a physician immediately. Excessive loss of body fluids in young children can lead to potentially fatal dehydration.

POSSIBLE SIDE EFFECTS
Rheaban is relatively free of serious side effects.

Ritalin®

GENERIC NAME
Methylphenidate hydrochloride.

PRODUCT CATEGORY
Central nervous system stimulant.

DOSAGE FORM
Tablets (5 mg, 10 mg, and 20 mg). It is also available in 20 mg SR (sustained-release) tablets.

WHY PRESCRIBED
It is used in the treatment of children diagnosed as having "attention deficit disorders"—previously known as minimal brain dysfunction (MBD). The cause of this condition is unknown. It is characterized by prolonged periods of impulsiveness, short attention span, emotional instability, easy distractibility, and moderate to severe hyperactivity.

CHILDREN'S DOSAGE
The usual starting dose is 5 milligrams given twice daily, before breakfast and lunch. This may be increased gradually in of 5 to 10 milligrams to a maximum daily dosage of 60 milligrams or until the desired response is achieved.

PRECAUTIONS AND WARNINGS
Ritalin should never be given to children under the age of six years. The drug should not be given to children with a history of convulsive seizures, because it may increase the frequency of attacks. Misuse of Ritalin can lead to psychological dependence on the drug.

POSSIBLE SIDE EFFECTS
The most common side effects are nervousness and the inability to fall asleep (insomnia). Some children may also experience loss of appetite (anorexia), headache, stomach upset, and dizziness.

Robicillin VK®

GENERIC NAME
Penicillin VK.

PRODUCT CATEGORY
Broad-spectrum antibiotic.

DOSAGE FORM
Tablets and oral solution.

WHY PRESCRIBED
It is used to treat a wide variety of bacterial infections.

CHILDREN'S DOSAGE
This depends on the severity of the infection, the type of bacteria involved, and the age and weight of the child. For example, the usual total daily dosage for infants and small children is 25,000 to 90,000 units (15 to 56 milligrams) per kilogram of body weight (1 kilogram = 2.2 pounds), given in three to six divided doses. Penicillin VK is not as easily affected by stomach acid as penicillin G. Thus, it is not necessary to take it on an empty stomach.

PRECAUTIONS AND WARNINGS
Penicillin should never be given to a child with a known allergy to it. Such hypersensitivity to the drug is greater in children who have experienced other allergies such as hay fever or hives (urticaria) or who have asthma.

Long-term use of any antibiotic may result in the development of a "superinfection"—the growth and multiplication in the body of fungi and other microorganisms that are not affected by the drug. Dispose of any remaining tablets or solution of penicillin once the course of therapy has been completed successfully.

POSSIBLE SIDE EFFECTS
The most commonly reported side effects are upset stomach, abdominal discomfort or pain, diarrhea, a black "hairy" tongue, and drug-induced fever. In children who are hypersensitive to the antibiotic, penicillin can cause a severe and potentially fatal allergic reaction (anaphylactic shock).

Robinul®

GENERIC NAME
Glycopyrrolate.

PRODUCT CATEGORY
Antispasmodic/anticholinergic.

DOSAGE FORM
Tablets (1 mg and 2 mg "Forte").

WHY PRESCRIBED
It is mainly used to decrease the frequency and severity of painful spasms of the stomach and intestines that are associated with various disorders of the gastrointestinal tract. It should not be used if the cause of abdominal pain is unknown.

CHILDREN'S DOSAGE
Robinul is not recommended for children under the age of twelve years. The dosage for older children will be determined by the physician, depending on the severity of the symptoms and the child's response to Robinul therapy.

PRECAUTIONS AND WARNINGS
Robinul should be used with caution in children with kidney or liver disease, heart disorders, or high blood pressure (hypertension).
　　The use of Robinul may interfere with the body's mechanism for sweating. Take care that the child is not subjected to high environmental temperatures while taking Robinul, because such exposure could lead to heat stroke or heat prostration.

POSSIBLE SIDE EFFECTS
Some children may experience dryness of the mouth, blurred vision, difficulty urinating, decreased sweating, rapid heartbeat (tachycardia), sensation of heartbeat (palpitations), nervousness, loss of taste, headache, drowsiness, dizziness, nausea, vomiting, constipation, and inability to sleep (insomnia).
　　Rarely, this class of drug (anticholinergic) may cause a drug-induced rash or hives (urticaria) or a severe allergic reaction (anaphylactic shock).

Robitet®

GENERIC NAME
Tetracycline.

PRODUCT CATEGORY
Antibacterial/antiamebic/antirickettsial.

DOSAGE FORM
Capsules.

WHY PRESCRIBED
It is used to treat infections caused by a wide range of microorganisms, including certain species of bacteria, protozoa, and rickettsiae (intermediate in size between bacteria and viruses).

CHILDREN'S DOSAGE
This depends on the child's weight. The usual total daily dosage of oral forms of tetracycline is 25 to 50 milligrams per kilogram of body weight (1 kilogram = 2.2 pounds), given in two to four equally divided doses. Tetracycline should not be given to children under the age of eight years, unless the physician determines that other antibiotics would be ineffective or inappropriate.

PRECAUTIONS AND WARNINGS
Tetracycline may cause permanent discoloration of the teeth if given to children under the age of eight years.

Do not give the child antacids while he or she is being treated with tetracycline, since this could interfere with the effectiveness of the antibiotic.

Tetracycline should be used with caution (if at all) in children with impaired liver or kidney function.

POSSIBLE SIDE EFFECTS
The most common side effects include nausea, vomiting, diarrhea, heartburn, flatulence (gas), and loss of appetite (anorexia). Tetracycline is capable of causing potentially serious side effects in some patients, including damage to the blood-forming tissues and severe generalized allergic reactions (anaphylactic shock).

Some children taking tetracycline may experience severe skin eruptions and rashes when exposed to strong sunlight. These exaggerated "sunburn reactions" usually disappear days or weeks after therapy with tetracycline has been discontinued.

Robitussin® (OTC)

GENERIC NAME
This product contains in each teaspoonful (5 ml) guaifenesin (100 mg) and alcohol (3.5 percent).

PRODUCT CATEGORY
Expectorant.

DOSAGE FORM
Syrup (wine color).

WHY USED
It is used to loosen phlegm and mucus in the air passages, thus making it easier to cough up and relieve congestion.

CHILDREN'S DOSAGE

Age of Child	Teaspoonfuls (5 ml) Every 4 Hours
12 years and over	2
6–11 years	1
2–5 years	½

PRECAUTIONS AND WARNINGS
Prolonged coughing (more than one week), especially if accompanied by fever or headache, may be a sign of a serious medical problem. In such cases, stop giving the child this product—or any other cough medicine—and consult a physician.

POSSIBLE SIDE EFFECTS
Used as directed, Robitussin is relatively free from side effects.

Robitussin-CF® (OTC)

GENERIC NAME
This product contains in each teaspoonful (5 ml) a combination of dextromethorphan hydrobromide (10 mg), phenylpropanolamine hydrochloride (12.5 mg), guaifenesin (100 mg), and alcohol (4.75 percent).

PRODUCT CATEGORY
Antitussive (cough suppressant)/expectorant.

DOSAGE FORM
Syrup (red color).

WHY USED
It is used to relieve coughing associated with the common cold, bronchitis, laryngitis, whooping cough (pertussis), influenza, measles, and chronic sinusitis.

CHILDREN'S DOSAGE

Age of Child	Teaspoonfuls (5 ml) Every 4 Hours
12 years and over	2
6–11 years	1
2–5 years	½

Do not give Robitussin-CF to children under the age of two years without the advice of a physician.

PRECAUTIONS AND WARNINGS
Do not give Robitussin-CF to a child with high blood pressure (hypertension), diabetes, or heart disease without medical approval.

Prolonged coughing, especially if it is accompanied by fever or headache, may be a sign of a serious medical problem. In such cases, stop giving the child any cough medicine and consult a physician.

POSSIBLE SIDE EFFECTS
The most commonly reported side effects include nausea, vomiting, dry mouth, nervousness, insomnia, and headache.

Romilar® Children's Cough Syrup (OTC)

GENERIC NAME
Dextromethorphan hydrobromide.

PRODUCT CATEGORY
Antitussive (cough suppressant).

DOSAGE FORM
Syrup (grape flavor).

WHY USED
It is used to relieve coughing associated with the common cold or acute bronchitis.

CHILDREN'S DOSAGE
Romilar is available without a doctor's prescription. Administer to children exactly as the label recommends.

PRECAUTIONS AND WARNINGS
This product should not be given to a child with a known hypersensitivity (allergy) to dextromethorphan. It also should not be used to treat coughing associated with a chronic disorder, such as asthma. Consult a physician if the child has a high fever, headache, rash, nausea, or vomiting, or if coughing produces blood or a thick yellowish mucus, which may be signs of a more serious underlying disorder.

POSSIBLE SIDE EFFECTS
When used as recommended, this product is unlikely to cause serious side effects. A skin rash, digestive upset, dizziness, or drowsiness may occur occasionally. Such side effects, if they occur, should be reported to the doctor.

Rondec®-DM Syrup

GENERIC NAME
This product contains in each teaspoonful (5 ml) carbinoxamine maleate (4 mg), and pseudoephedrine hydrochloride (60 mg).

PRODUCT CATEGORY
Antihistamine/decongestant.

DOSAGE FORM
Syrup and tablets.

WHY PRESCRIBED
It is used for the relief of symptoms of the common cold, bronchitis, and postnasal drip.

CHILDREN'S DOSAGE
This depends on the age of the child, the severity of the symptoms, and the child's response to the drug. The usual dosage of the syrup form of the drug for children between the ages of eighteen months and five years is one-half teaspoonful (2.5 ml), given four times daily. Children age six years and over receive one teaspoonful (5 ml) four times daily. Children between one month and eighteen months of age are usually given oral drops in amounts prescribed by the doctor.

PRECAUTIONS AND WARNINGS
Rondec-DM Syrup and drops should be used with caution (if at all) in children with high blood pressure (hypertension), heart disease, asthma, thyroid disease, or diabetes.

POSSIBLE SIDE EFFECTS
The most commonly reported side effects include sedation, dizziness, blurred vision, headache, nausea, vomiting, dryness of the mouth, nervousness, difficulty urinating, and abdominal discomfort or stomach upset. The antihistamine ingredient may cause excitability in some children, especially if larger than prescribed doses are used.

St. Joseph® Aspirin for Children (OTC)

GENERIC NAME
Aspirin (81 mg).

PRODUCT CATEGORY
Analgesic/antipyretic anti-inflammatory.

DOSAGE FORM
Chewable tablets (orange flavor)

WHY USED
It is used to relieve symptoms of pain (analgesic effect), fever (antipyretic effect), and redness and swelling (anti-inflammatory effect) associated with headache, the common cold, muscular aches and pains, toothache, and various forms of arthritis.

CHILDREN'S DOSAGE

Age of Child	Tablets Every 4 Hours, if Needed
12–23 months	1½
2–3 years	2
4–5 years	3
6–8 years	4
9–10 years	5
11 years	6
12 or more years	8

Do not give a child the recommended dosage more than a maximum of five times a day. Larger doses may be prescribed by a physician.

PRECAUTIONS AND WARNINGS
Consult a physician before giving aspirin to children, including teenagers, who may have or may be recovering from influenza or chicken pox. Also, check with a physician before giving aspirin to a child with bleeding problems, a stomach disorder, asthma, or allergies. Children should not take aspirin for more than five consecutive days or exceed the dosage on the label, unless under medical supervision.

To minimize stomach irritation, always give the child aspirin with food or with water, milk, or fruit juice.

If fever persists for more than three days, or returns, consult a physician. If the child experiences high fever, headache, nausea and vomiting, or a sore throat, discontinue use of the drug and contact a physician.

St. Joseph® Aspirin for Children (OTC) (Continued)

POSSIBLE SIDE EFFECTS
The most common side effects are nausea, vomiting, and stomach pain. Children who are allergic to aspirin may experience itching, skin rash, shortness of breath, and wheezing. Aspirin also may cause digestive tract bleeding.

ASPIRIN ALERT
Consult your doctor when giving aspirin products to reduce fever. The U.S. Department of Health and Human Services warns that giving aspirin to a child with fever increases the risk of Reye's syndrome. Read the notice on pp. 15 ff.

St. Joseph® Aspirin-Free for Children (OTC)

GENERIC NAME
Acetaminophen.

PRODUCT CATEGORY
Analgesic (pain reliever)/antipyretic (fever reducer).

DOSAGE FORM
Chewable tablets (80 mg), elixir (160 mg per 5 ml teaspoonful), and fruit-flavored drops (80 mg per 0.8 ml dropperful).

WHY USED
It is used to relieve the symptoms of fever and minor aches and pains associated with the common cold and flu.

CHILDREN'S DOSAGE

Age of Child	Tablets Every 4 Hours, if Needed
12–23 months	1½
2–3 years	2
4–5 years	3
6–8 years	4
9–10 years	5
11 years	6
12 years and over	8

St. Joseph Aspirin-Free drops or elixir may be prescribed by a physician in specific doses for children younger than one year. Do not exceed five doses daily for a child of any age.

PRECAUTIONS AND WARNINGS
Do not give a child acetaminophen for more than five consecutive days. If a fever continues for more than three days, consult a physician. If the symptoms continue, or new ones develop, contact the doctor. If the child develops a sore throat, high fever, headache, or nausea and vomiting, discontinue use of the product and consult a physician. Do not give a child any other medication containing acetaminophen at the same time without the advice of a doctor.

POSSIBLE SIDE EFFECTS
When used as recommended, side effects are relatively uncommon. Liver damage may result when larger than recommended doses are used or acetaminophen is taken for prolonged periods. Other occasional adverse effects may include rashes, urticaria (hives), drug-induced fever, and blood changes.

St. Joseph® Cough Syrup for Children (OTC)

GENERIC NAME
Dextromethorphan hydrobromide (7.5 mg per 5 ml teaspoonful).

PRODUCT CATEGORY
Antitussive (cough suppressant).

DOSAGE FORM
Syrup (cherry flavor).

WHY USED
It is used to relieve coughing associated with the common cold and flu.

CHILDREN'S DOSAGE

Age of Child	Teaspoonfuls (5 ml) Every 6 to 8 Hours
2–5 years	1
6–11 years	2
12 years and over	4

Do not exceed four doses daily. Do not give St. Joseph Cough Syrup to children under the age of two years without the advice of a physician.

PRECAUTIONS AND WARNINGS
Prolonged coughing, especially if accompanied by a fever or headache, may be a sign of a serious medical problem. In such cases, stop giving the child this product and consult a physician.

POSSIBLE SIDE EFFECTS
Used as directed, St. Joseph Cough Syrup for Children is relatively free from adverse effects. Rarely reported side effects from the use of dextromethorphan include dizziness, drowsiness, digestive disorders, and skin rashes.

Scabene®

GENERIC NAME
Lindane (1 percent).

PRODUCT CATEGORY
Parasiticide (antiparasitic)/ovicide (destroys eggs).

DOSAGE FORM
Lotion (liquid for external use only). A shampoo also is available.

WHY PRESCRIBED
It is used to eradicate infestations of scabies ("the itch"), caused by an itch mite (*Sarcoptes scabies*) that burrows in the skin of humans. The shampoo is also used in the treatment of infestations of crab lice (pediculosis pubis).

CHILDREN'S DOSAGE
The lotion is applied to dry skin and allowed to remain for eight to twelve hours before removing the chemical with a thorough washing of the treated skin. The product should not be allowed to come into contact with the eyes or skin abrasions or cuts. It is recommended that the person applying the product wear rubber gloves during application.

PRECAUTIONS AND WARNINGS
Lindane can penetrate the human skin and cause adverse effects to the central nervous system. Special care should be taken in the use of the product on infants and children as they are more likely to suffer adverse effects from skin absorption than adults. Avoid any unnecessary skin contact, and do not use more of the product than is needed. Scabene is for external use only.

POSSIBLE SIDE EFFECTS
Most side effects involve central nervous system stimulation and may range from dizziness to convulsions. Pruritus (itching) may occur after use of Scabene but it is usually not a sign of treatment failure and treatment should not be repeated unless living mites are found. Some children may develop an eczema-like skin irritation as a result of the application of lindane to the skin.

Septra®

GENERIC NAME
This product contains trimethoprim and sulfamethoxazole.

PRODUCT CATEGORY
Antibacterial (combination including a sulfonamide).

DOSAGE FORM
Liquid (oral suspension). Tablets are also available.

WHY PRESCRIBED
It is mainly used in children to treat bacterial infections of the urinary tract (kidneys and bladder) and those that involve the middle ear (acute otitis media).

CHILDREN'S DOSAGE

Body Weight	Teaspoonfuls (5 ml) Every 12 Hours	Tablets
22 lb (10 kg)	1	½
44 lb (20 kg)	2	1
66 lb (30 kg)	3	1½
88 lb (40 kg)	4	2

PRECAUTIONS AND WARNINGS
Stop giving Septra to a child who develops a skin rash, sore throat, or jaundice (yellowness of the skin), and consult a physician immediately.

Have the child drink plenty of water while taking this drug to help prevent the formation of crystals of Septra in the kidneys.

Septra should not be given to infants under the age of two months.

Septra should never be used to treat a strep throat.

Before giving this drug to a child, be sure the physician is aware of any severe allergies, bronchial asthma, or kidney or liver disease the child may have or have had in the past.

POSSIBLE SIDE EFFECTS
The most common side effects experienced by some children taking Septra include headache, nausea, vomiting, diarrhea, stomach pain or discomfort, and ringing in the ears (tinnitus).

Septra contains a sulfa drug (sulfamethoxazole), which in some children may cause a potentially serious allergic reaction.

Sinarest® Tablets (OTC)

GENERIC NAME
This product contains a combination of acetaminophen (325 or 500 mg), chlorpheniramine maleate (2 mg), and phenylpropanolamine hydrochloride (18.7 mg).

PRODUCT CATEGORY
Analgesic/antihistamine/decongestant.

DOSAGE FORM
Tablets (regular with 325 mg acetaminophen and extra strength with 500 mg acetaminophen).

WHY USED
It is used to relieve the symptoms of pain, congestion, and discomfort associated with the common cold, sinusitis, and allergic rhinitis (runny nose).

CHILDREN'S DOSAGE
Dosages for children under six years of age should be individualized by a physician. For children between six and twelve years of age, the usual recommended dose is one regular strength tablet every four hours, but not more than four tablets a day. Extra strength tablets should not be given children under the age of twelve years. For older children, the recommended dose is two extra strength tablets every six hours, but not more than eight tablets a day.

PRECAUTIONS AND WARNINGS
This product should not be given to a child with a known hypersensitivity (allergy) to any of the ingredients. It should be used with caution (if at all) in children with high blood pressure, heart disease, thyroid disease, or diabetes. Consult a physician if the child is taking any other medication that might react adversely with the ingredients in Sinarest. Do not use Sinarest tablets for more than ten consecutive days.

POSSIBLE SIDE EFFECTS
The most serious reported side effect, liver damage, is usually the result of taking larger than recommended amounts of the medicine. Other possible side effects include drowsiness, excitability, nervousness, and dizziness.

Sinex® (OTC)

GENERIC NAME
This product contains a combination of phenylephrine hydrochloride (0.5 percent), cetylpyridinium chloride (0.04 percent), and various aromatics, including menthol, camphor, eucalyptol, and methyl salicylate.

PRODUCT CATEGORY
Decongestant.

DOSAGE FORM
Nasal spray.

WHY USED
It is used to relieve the symptoms of nasal congestion (stuffy nose) associated with head colds, hay fever, sinusitis, and respiratory allergies.

CHILDREN'S DOSAGE
This product is available without a doctor's prescription. However, it is not recommended for use in children under the age of six years without the advice of a physician. Otherwise, use the product as directed by instructions on the label.

PRECAUTIONS AND WARNINGS
If the symptoms continue or worsen, discontinue use of the product and consult a physician.

POSSIBLE SIDE EFFECTS
Although side effects are uncommon when the product is used as directed, the phenylephrine ingredient may be a cause of headaches, excitability, and heartbeat abnormalities in some sensitive children, particularly if larger than recommended doses are used.

SK-Ampicillin®

GENERIC NAME
Ampicillin.

PRODUCT CATEGORY
Broad-spectrum antibiotic (semisynthetic penicillin).

DOSAGE FORM
Capsules and oral suspension.

WHY PRESCRIBED
This product is used to treat a wide range of bacterial infections in children, including those that involve the middle ear (otitis media), stomach and intestines (gastrointestinal tract), urinary tract, respiratory tract, the membranes that cover the brain (meningitis), and the skin.

CHILDREN'S DOSAGE
This depends largely on the severity of the infection and the age and body weight of the child. The site of infection can also affect the dosage. For example, the usual dosage for children with an infection of the respiratory tract is 250 milligrams every six hours. However, if the child weighs less than 20 kilograms (44 pounds), the total daily dosage may be 50 milligrams per kilogram of body weight (1 kilogram = 2.2 pounds), given in equally divided doses every six or eight hours. If it is kept refrigerated, ampicillin suspension should remain stable for two weeks.

PRECAUTIONS AND WARNINGS
Ampicillin should never be given to a child who is known to be allergic to it or to penicillin. Adverse reactions are more likely if the child has experienced other allergies such as hay fever or hives (urticaria) or has asthma.

POSSIBLE SIDE EFFECTS
The most common side effects are diarrhea and skin rashes. Some children may also experience nausea and vomiting. More serious side effects are relatively uncommon.

SK-Erythromycin®

GENERIC NAME
Erythromycin stearate.

PRODUCT CATEGORY
Antibiotic.

DOSAGE FORM
Tablets.

WHY PRESCRIBED
SK-Erythromycin is used to treat mild to moderate bacterial infections, especially when the child is known to be allergic to penicillin or when the bacteria do not respond to penicillin.

CHILDREN'S DOSAGE
The dosage depends largely on the severity of the infection and the child's age and body weight. The usual daily dosage is 30 to 50 milligrams per kilogram of body weight (1 kilogram = 2.2 pounds), given in divided doses three or four times a day. In treating particularly severe infections, the physician may double this dose.

PRECAUTIONS AND WARNINGS
Children should take SK-Erythromycin at the times and in the exact amounts prescribed by their physician. Taking more than the prescribed amount can cause stomach discomfort, nausea, vomiting, and diarrhea.

Long-term use of any antibiotic may result in the development of a "superinfection"—the growth and multiplication in the body of fungi and other microorganisms that are not affected by the drug.

POSSIBLE SIDE EFFECTS
Erythromycin is a relatively safe antibiotic, and serious side effects are uncommon. Allergic (hypersensitivity) reactions are usually mild and include hives (urticaria) and rashes. Because erythromycin can stimulate digestive tract activity, the child may experience nausea, diarrhea, or stomach cramps.

SK-Penicillin VK®

GENERIC NAME
Penicillin VK.

PRODUCT CATEGORY
Broad-spectrum antibiotic.

DOSAGE FORM
Tablets and oral solution.

WHY PRESCRIBED
It is used to treat a wide variety of bacterial infections.

CHILDREN'S DOSAGE
This depends on the severity of the infection, the type of bacteria involved, and the age and body weight of the child. For example, the total daily dosage for infants and small children is 25,000 to 90,000 units (15 to 56 mg) per kilogram of body weight (1 kilogram = 2.2 pounds), given in three to six divided doses. Penicillin VK is not as easily affected by stomach acids as is penicillin G. Thus, it is not necessary to take it on an empty stomach.

PRECAUTIONS AND WARNINGS
Penicillin should never be given to a child with a known allergy to it. Such hypersensitivity to the drug is greater in children who have experienced other allergies such as hay fever or hives (urticaria) or who have asthma.

Long-term use of any antibiotic may result in development of a "superinfection"—the growth and multiplication in the body of fungi and other microorganisms that are not affected by the drug. Dispose of any remaining tablets or oral solution once the course of therapy has been completed successfully.

POSSIBLE SIDE EFFECTS
The most commonly reported side effects are upset stomach, abdominal discomfort or pain, diarrhea, a black "hairy" tongue, and drug-induced fever. In children who are hypersensitive to the antibiotic, penicillin can cause a severe and potentially fatal allergic reaction (anaphylactic shock).

SK-Pramine®

GENERIC NAME
Imipramine hydrochloride.

PRODUCT CATEGORY
Antidepressant/antienuretic.

DOSAGE FORM
Tablets.

WHY PRESCRIBED
It is used to relieve the symptoms of depression and also in the therapy of children over the age of five years who have bed-wetting problems.

CHILDREN'S DOSAGE
The product is not recommended for the treatment of children with conditions other than nocturnal enuresis (nighttime bed-wetting). It is intended for use only in children six years of age and older. The exact daily dosage is determined by the prescribing physician, who usually establishes the smallest daily dose that will be effective in reducing enuresis.

PRECAUTIONS AND WARNINGS
SK-Pramine is not intended for prolonged uses and it is recommended that a drug-free period be tried after some success has been achieved in controlling enuresis. The product should not be taken at the same time as certain other types of drugs, particularly those that contain epinephrine, without the advice of a physician. Because imipramine may affect heart function, the doctor may order an electrocardiogram for the child before prescribing a larger than minimum dosage. The child should avoid excessive exposure to sunlight while taking imipramine because the drug may cause an adverse reaction in sunlight.

POSSIBLE SIDE EFFECTS
Among the more commonly reported side effects of imipramine are headache, insomnia, dry mouth, unpleasant taste, fatigue, weakness, nausea, indigestion, and constipation or diarrhea.

SK-Tetracycline®

GENERIC NAME
Tetracycline.

PRODUCT CATEGORY
Antibacterial/antiamebic/antirickettsial.

DOSAGE FORM
Capsules and oral suspension.

WHY PRESCRIBED
It is used to treat infections caused by a wide range of microorganisms, including certain species of bacteria, protozoa, and rickettsiae (intermediate in size between bacteria and viruses).

CHILDREN'S DOSAGE
This depends mainly on the child's weight. The usual total daily dosage of oral forms of tetracycline is 25 to 50 milligrams per kilogram of body weight (1 kilogram = 2.2 pounds), given in two to four equally divided doses. Tetracycline should not be given to children under the age of eight, unless the physician determines that other antibiotics would be ineffective or inappropriate.

PRECAUTIONS AND WARNINGS
Tetracycline may cause permanent discoloration of the teeth if given to children under the age of eight years.

Do not give the child antacids while he or she is being treated with tetracycline, since this could interfere with the effectiveness of the antibiotic.

Tetracycline should be used with caution (if at all) in children with impaired liver or kidney function.

POSSIBLE SIDE EFFECTS
The most common side effects include nausea, vomiting, diarrhea, heartburn, flatulence (gas), and loss of appetite (anorexia). Tetracycline is capable of causing potentially serious side effects in some patients, including damage to the blood-forming tissues and a severe generalized allergic reaction (anaphylactic shock).

Some children taking tetracycline may experience severe skin eruptions and rashes when exposed to strong sunlight. These exaggerated "sunburn reactions" usually disappear days or weeks after therapy with tetracycline has been discontinued.

Slo-Bid®

GENERIC NAME
Theophylline.

PRODUCT CATEGORY
Bronchodilator.

DOSAGE FORM
Capsules (timed-release Gyrocaps®).

WHY PRESCRIBED
It is used to prevent and relieve symptoms of asthma and bronchospasm associated with chronic bronchitis.

CHILDREN'S DOSAGE
This product is not recommended for use in children under the age of six years. The exact dosage varies with the age and lean body weight of the child and the frequency of doses. The physician will individualize the dosage according to the needs and response of the child. The physician also may adjust the dosage after an initial period of drug use.

PRECAUTIONS AND WARNINGS
This product should not be given to a child who has a known hypersensitivity (allergy) to theophylline. The drug should not be given to a child taking other medications containing theophylline or related substances. Caution should be used in giving the child caffeine beverages, including colas, or large amounts of chocolate at the same time as theophylline medications. It should not be given to a child with heart disease, hypertension (high blood pressure), liver disease, or thyroid disease without the advice of a physician.

POSSIBLE SIDE EFFECTS
Among side effects commonly reported are headache, irritability, nervousness, restlessness, insomnia, nausea, vomiting, and stomach pain. Less frequently observed side effects include dizziness or lightheadedness, skin rash or hives (urticaria), diarrhea, and appetite loss (anorexia).

Slo-Phyllin®

GENERIC NAME
Theophylline.

PRODUCT CATEGORY
Bronchodilator.

DOSAGE FORM
Syrup, tablets, and capsules (timed-release Gyrocaps®).

WHY PRESCRIBED
It is used to prevent and relieve symptoms of asthma and bronchospasm associated with chronic bronchitis.

CHILDREN'S DOSAGE
This product is not recommended for use in infants under the age of six months. The timed-release form of the drug is not recommended for children under the age of six years. The exact dosage is determined by a number of factors, including the age and *lean* body weight of the child, the frequency of doses, the form of the drug used, and whether the condition is acute or chronic. The prescribing physician will individualize the dose and may adjust it upward or downward according to the needs and response of the child.

PRECAUTIONS AND WARNING
Theophylline should not be given to a child who is already taking a similar type of medication. It should be used with caution (if at all) in a child with heart disease, hypertension (high blood pressure), liver disease, or thyroid disease. Because theophylline may irritate the digestive tract, it should not be given to a child with peptic ulcers except with the advice of a physician. A child taking theophylline drugs should not be given caffeine beverages, including colas, or large amounts of chocolate, without the approval of a physician.

POSSIBLE SIDE EFFECTS
Most side effects are the result of giving a child larger than prescribed doses of theophylline and may include nausea, vomiting (sometimes with bloody vomit), diarrhea, abdominal pain, headache, irritability, restlessness, insomnia, muscle twitching, rapid breathing, rapid heartbeat (tachycardia), and sensation of heartbeat (palpitations).

Sodium Sulamyd®

GENERIC NAME
Sulfacetamide sodium.

PRODUCT CATEGORY
Ophthalmic (eye) preparation/antibacterial.

DOSAGE FORM
Eyedrops and opthalmic ointment.

WHY PRESCRIBED
It is used in the treatment of conjunctivitis, ulcer of the cornea, and other bacterial infections of the eye.

CHILDREN'S DOSAGE
This depends on the severity of the infection. The physician will determine the dosage based on the specific needs and therapeutic response of the child.

PRECAUTIONS AND WARNINGS
Do not allow the eyedropper to touch anything that may contaminate it, and do not let the dropper touch the eye.

POSSIBLE SIDE EFFECTS
The most commonly reported side effects are local irritation and temporary stinging or burning as the drug is applied. Allergic reactions are relatively rare. If an allergic reaction occurs, stop giving the drug and consult a doctor.

Solfoton®

GENERIC NAME
Phenobarbital.

PRODUCT CATEGORY
Sedative/anticonvulsant (barbiturate).

DOSAGE FORM
Tablets and capsules.

WHY PRESCRIBED
It is used to calm anxiety and help induce sleep (sedative action). It also may be used alone or with other drugs to prevent and control convulsions or seizures (anticonvulsant or antiepileptic action).

CHILDREN'S DOSAGE
This depends on the condition being treated and the body weight of the child. For example, the usual dosage to control convulsions may be 16 to 48 milligrams two to three times daily. For sedation of children, the usual total daily dosage is 6 milligrams per kilogram of body weight, given in divided doses three times a day.

PRECAUTIONS AND WARNINGS
Phenobarbital may be habit-forming. Children with an inborn (hereditary) error of metabolism known as porphyria must not take phenobarbital or other barbiturates. The drug should be used with caution (if at all) in children with a disease of the liver or kidneys.

POSSIBLE SIDE EFFECTS
The most commonly reported side effects are drowsiness (which is a therapeutic effect when phenobarbital is used as a sedative), dizziness, depression, vomiting, diarrhea, impaired breathing, and allergic reactions such as skin rashes.

Overdosage with phenobarbital can be fatal.

Somophyllin® -T

GENERIC NAME
Theophylline.

PRODUCT CATEGORY
Bronchodilator.

DOSAGE FORM
Capsules.

WHY PRESCRIBED
It is used to prevent and relieve the symptoms of asthma and bronchospasm associated with chronic bronchitis.

CHILDREN'S DOSAGE
The exact dosage is individualized according to the age and *lean* body weight of the child, and other factors which may include whether the condition is acute or chronic, and the frequency of doses. Also, the prescribing physician usually adjusts the dosage upward or downward after an initial period of therapy according to the needs and response of the child to the drug.

PRECAUTIONS AND WARNINGS
Do not give this drug to a child who is already taking a medication containing theophylline or a related substance. Use caution in giving the child caffeine beverages, including colas, or large amounts of chocolate while also giving theophylline. Do not give this product to a child with heart disease, thyroid disease, hypertension (high blood pressure), or impaired liver or kidney function. Because theophylline can irritate the digestive tract of some individuals, it should not be given to a child with peptic ulcers without the advice and supervision of a physician.

POSSIBLE SIDE EFFECTS
Most common side effects resulting from the use of theophylline are due to larger than prescribed doses and may include nausea, vomiting (sometimes with bloody vomit), abdominal pain, diarrhea, headache, irritability, restlessness, insomnia, muscle twitching, rapid breathing, rapid heartbeat (tachycardia), and sensation of heartbeat (palpitations).

Sterapred®

GENERIC NAME
Prednisone.

PRODUCT CATEGORY
Corticosteroid (synthetic glucocorticoid)/anti-inflammatory.

DOSAGE FORM
Tablets.

WHY PRESCRIBED
It is used in the treatment of a wide variety of inflammatory and allergic conditions. Sterapred is often used in combination with other corticosteroids in treating disorders of the adrenal glands, to replace hormones normally produced by these glands.

CHILDREN'S DOSAGE
This depends on the type and severity of the condition being treated and the response of the child to Sterapred therapy. The physician will individualize the dosage requirements.

PRECAUTIONS AND WARNINGS
Children should not be vaccinated against smallpox or be subjected to other immunization procedures while using corticosteroid therapy. As Sterapred may interact with aspirin and many other prescription and nonprescription drugs, resulting in adverse effects, the doctor should be consulted about giving the child any additional medications while taking this product. Prednisone products may affect response of the child to surgery, injury, or illness for up to two years after the drug has been discontinued. Thus, any doctor providing care for the child in the next two years should be advised of the child's previous use of the drug.

POSSIBLE SIDE EFFECTS
All drugs in the general class of corticosteroids, such as Sterapred, are capable of causing a wide range of adverse reactions. These are largely related to the dosage and the duration of therapy. Among the reported side effects are suppressed growth in children; accumulation of fatty deposits around the face, neck, or abdomen; nervousness; decreased bone density (osteoporosis); increased susceptibility to infection; water retention, resulting in swelling of tissues (edema); euphoria; insomnia; skin changes, and increased susceptibility to bruising.

Sudafed® (OTC)

GENERIC NAME
Pseudoephedrine hydrochloride.

PRODUCT CATEGORY
Decongestant.

DOSAGE FORM
Tablets (30 mg) and syrup (30 mg per 5 ml teaspoonful).

WHY USED
It is used to relieve the symptoms of hay fever (allergic rhinitis) and the common cold. These include stuffy nose (nasal congestion), congested sinuses, and (when under medical supervision) congestion and blockage of the eustachian tube—the canal between the middle ear and the upper part of the throat that equalizes air pressure on either side of the eardrum.

CHILDREN'S DOSAGE
Children between the ages of two and five years should be given only the syrup form of Sudafed. The usual dosage is one-half teaspoonful (2.5 ml) every four hours, up to a maximum of four doses within a 24-hour period. The usual dosage for children between the ages of six and twelve is one teaspoonful (5 ml) or one tablet every four hours. Children age twelve and over may be given two teaspoonfuls every four hours up to a maximum of four doses a day.

Do not give Sudafed to a child under the age of two years without medical supervision.

PRECAUTIONS AND WARNINGS
Sudafed should be used with caution in children with high blood pressure (hypertension), heart disease, diabetes, difficulty urinating, or thyroid disease, and then only with the advice and supervision of a physician.

POSSIBLE SIDE EFFECTS
The most commonly reported side effects include nervousness, dizziness, nausea, sleeplessness, and headache. Should these occur while the child is not under medical care, reduce the dosage or discontinue use of the product and consult a physician.

Sumycin®

GENERIC NAME
Tetracycline.

PRODUCT CATEGORY
Antibacterial/antiamebic/antirickettsial.

DOSAGE FORM
Tablets, capsules, and oral suspension.

WHY PRESCRIBED
It is used to treat infections caused by a wide range of microorganisms, including certain species of bacteria, protozoa, and rickettsiae (intermediate in size between bacteria and viruses).

CHILDREN'S DOSAGE
This depends on the child's body weight. The usual total daily dosage of oral forms of tetracycline is 25 to 50 milligrams per kilogram of body weight (1 kilogram = 2.2 pounds), given in two to four equally divided doses. Tetracycline should not be given to children under the age of eight years unless the physician considers that other antibiotics would be ineffective or inappropriate.

PRECAUTIONS AND WARNINGS
Tetracycline may cause permanent discoloration of the teeth if given to children under the age of eight years.

Do not give the child antacids while he or she is being treated with tetracycline, since this could interfere with the effectiveness of the antibiotic.

Tetracycline should be used with caution (if at all) in children with impaired liver or kidney function.

POSSIBLE SIDE EFFECTS
The most common side effects include nausea, vomiting, gas (flatulence), heartburn, diarrhea, and loss of appetite (anorexia). Tetracycline is capable of causing potentially more serious side effects in some patients, including damage to the blood-forming tissues and a severe generalized allergic reaction (anaphylactic shock).

Some children taking tetracycline may experience severe skin eruptions and rashes when exposed to strong sunlight. These exaggerated "sunburn reactions" usually disappear days or weeks after therapy with tetracycline has been discontinued.

Sustaire®

GENERIC NAME
Theophylline.

PRODUCT CATEGORY
Bronchodilator.

DOSAGE FORM
Tablets (sustained-release).

WHY PRESCRIBED
It is used to prevent and relieve symptoms of asthma and bronchospasm associated with chronic bronchitis.

CHILDREN'S DOSAGE
This depends on several factors, including the age and *lean* body weight of the child, the frequency of doses, and whether the condition is acute or chronic. The physician will individualize the dosage, with upward or downward adjustments according to the needs and response of the child to the therapy.

PRECAUTIONS AND WARNINGS
This product should not be given to a child with a known hypersensitivity (allergy) to theophylline. It also should not be given to a child who is already taking a medication that contains theophylline or a related substance. Caution should be used in giving caffeine beverages, including colas, or large amounts of chocolate to children taking theophylline medications. It should not be given to a child with heart disease, thyroid disease, hypertension (high blood pressure), or impaired liver function without the advice and supervision of a physician. Theophylline may irritate the digestive tract of some children.

POSSIBLE SIDE EFFECTS
The most commonly reported side effects are nausea and vomiting (sometimes with bloody vomit), abdominal pain, diarrhea, headache, irritability, restlessness, insomnia, muscle twitching, rapid breathing, rapid heartbeat (tachycardia), and sensation of heartbeat (palpitations).

Synalar®

GENERIC NAME
Fluocinolone acetonide.

PRODUCT CATEGORY
Anti-inflammatory (synthetic corticosteroid).

DOSAGE FORM
Cream, ointment, and solution.

WHY PRESCRIBED
It is used to treat various inflammatory disorders of the skin that are responsive to corticosteroids.

CHILDREN'S DOSAGE
The physician will give specific directions for use. In general, the ointment form of Synalar is used to treat dry or scaly areas of inflamed skin. If the inflamed area is moist, the cream or solution forms of the drug are usually best. Apply three or four times daily, or as instructed.

PRECAUTIONS AND WARNINGS
Do not apply Synalar to areas of the child's skin that are infected. Not only does the drug have no beneficial effect on bacterial or fungal infections, but it may cause the disease to spread to nearby areas of healthy skin.

If Synalar causes local irritation of the skin, or if the inflammation seems to worsen, discontinue the use of the drug and consult the physician.

POSSIBLE SIDE EFFECTS
The most commonly reported side effects include itching, dry skin, skin eruptions, and a burning sensation at the site of drug application.

More serious side effects may occur if Synalar is applied to extensive areas of skin and left on for prolonged periods. However, this is unlikely if the child is under close medical supervision and the physician's instructions are closely followed.

Talwin® Nx

GENERIC NAME
This product contains a combination of pentazocine hydrochloride (50 mg) and naloxone hydrochloride (0.5 mg).

PRODUCT CATEGORY
Analgesic (pain reliever).

DOSAGE FORM
Tablets.

WHY PRESCRIBED
It is used for the relief of moderate to severe pain.

CHILDREN'S DOSAGE
Talwin should not be given to children under the age of twelve years. For older children, the usual dosage is one tablet (50 mg) every three or four hours. The physician may double this amount to control particularly severe pain. The total daily dosage of Talwin should not exceed 600 milligrams.

PRECAUTIONS AND WARNINGS
Talwin should be given with extreme caution (if at all) to children with convulsive disorders, bronchial asthma, or kidney or liver impairment.

Do not give children any other drugs at the same time as Talwin without the knowledge and approval of the doctor.

POSSIBLE SIDE EFFECTS
The most commonly reported side effects include stomach upset, nausea, vomiting, abdominal cramps, constipation, diarrhea, dry mouth, dizziness, headache, lightheadedness, sedation, irritability, sleeping difficulty, and altered taste.

Some patients may also experience flushing, blurred vision, hallucinations, difficulty breathing, changes in blood pressure, tingling in arms and legs, rapid heartbeat (tachycardia), drug-induced skin rashes, and impairment of blood-forming tissues.

Tedral®

GENERIC NAME
This product contains a combination of ephedrine hydrochloride, theophylline, phenobarbital, and alcohol (15 percent in the elixir).

PRODUCT CATEGORY
Bronchodilator/anti-asthmatic.

DOSAGE FORM
Elixir, oral suspension, and tablets.

WHY PRESCRIBED
It is used to relieve the symptoms of wheezing and shortness of breath in children with bronchial asthma.

CHILDREN'S DOSAGE
Because this product contains phenobarbital (a potentially habit-forming drug), a doctor's prescription may be required in certain states that prohibit over-the-counter (OTC) sales of phenobarbital. In such cases, the prescribing physician will determine the appropriate dosage for an individual child. Severe forms of asthma will require more effective prescription drugs to control attacks. In areas where the drug is available without a prescription, administer to the child exactly as the label recommends.

PRECAUTIONS AND WARNINGS
Do not give Tedral to a child unless a medical diagnosis of asthma has been made. A child with symptoms of asthma should be examined by a physician before any medication is given. Do not give this product to children with heart disease, hypertension (high blood pressure), or diabetes unless approved by a physician.

The phenobarbital in Tedral can be habit-forming, especially if it is taken in large amounts for prolonged periods.

If the child's symptoms fail to improve, seek medical attention at once.

POSSIBLE SIDE EFFECTS
Used as directed, Tedral is relatively free from side effects. Some children may experience nervousness, restlessness, and sleeplessness. Should any of these side effects occur, stop giving the child Tedral and consult a physician. Sensitivity to phenobarbital may result from an inherited pigment disorder known as porphyria.

Tegopen®

GENERIC NAME
Cloxacillin sodium.

PRODUCT CATEGORY
Antibiotic (synthetic penicillin).

DOSAGE FORM
Liquid (oral solution) and capsules.

WHY PRESCRIBED
It is mainly used to treat children with specific types of bacterial infection (those caused by strains of bacteria that are able to destroy penicillin).

CHILDREN'S DOSAGE
This depends on the child's body weight and the severity of the infection. The usual daily dosage for children who weigh at least 20 kilograms (44 pounds) is 250 milligrams every six hours. For children who weigh less than 20 kilograms, the usual total daily dosage is 50 milligrams per kilogram of body weight (1 kilogram = 2.2 pounds), given in equally divided doses every six hours. In treating particularly severe infections, the physician may double this amount.

PRECAUTIONS AND WARNINGS
Tegopen should not be given to a child with a known allergy to it or to other forms of penicillin. Such sensitivity to the drug is greater in children who have experienced other allergies such as hay fever or hives (urticaria) or who have asthma.

Long-term use of any antibiotic may result in development of a "superinfection"—the growth and multiplication in the body of fungi and other microorganisms that are unaffected by the drug. Dispose of any remaining solution or capsules of Tegopen once the course of therapy has been successfully completed.

POSSIBLE SIDE EFFECTS
The most commonly reported side effects include nausea, abdominal discomfort, and diarrhea. In children who are hypersensitive to the antibiotic, Tegopen is capable of causing a severe and potentially fatal allergic reaction (anaphylactic shock).

Tegretol®

GENERIC NAME
Carbamazepine.

PRODUCT CATEGORY
Anticonvulsant (antiepileptic).

DOSAGE FORM
Tablets and chewable tablets.

WHY PRESCRIBED
It is used mainly to prevent or control grand mal epielptic seizures, temporal lobe and other partial seizures, and mixed seizure patterns. (It is not used for petit mal seizures.) Its use is generally restricted to patients who have failed to respond satisfactorily to other drugs, such as phenobarbital or phenytoin.

CHILDREN'S DOSAGE
Tegretol is a potent and potentially toxic drug. It is not recommended for children under six years of age. The physician will adjust the dosage according to the needs and response of the child. Once Tegretol has been found to be effective, a daily maintenance dosage for children between the ages of six and twelve years is usually 400 to 800 milligrams, given in divided doses. For children over the age of twelve, the daily maintenance dosage is usually 800 to 1,200 milligrams, given in divided doses. The physician will usually prescribe the minimum amount that is effective.

PRECAUTIONS AND WARNINGS
Tegretol must be taken as prescribed by the physician. Before the drug is prescribed, and periodically while therapy is underway, blood tests are required to ensure that blood-forming tissues are not affected by the product.

Discontinue giving the child this drug and consult the physician immediately if early signs of adverse effects are observed. These include fever, sore throat, mouth sores, or unusual bruising or bleeding.

POSSIBLE SIDE EFFECTS
Tegretol may cause serious impairment of blood-forming tissues in some children. Less severe side effects reported with the use of Tegretol include drowsiness, unsteadiness, dizziness, nausea, and vomiting. These effects are usually noted during the early stages of therapy and may disappear once the dosage has been adjusted.

Teldrin® (OTC)

GENERIC NAME
Chlorpheniramine maleate.

PRODUCT CATEGORY
Antihistamine.

DOSAGE FORM
Timed-release capsules (8 mg and maximum strength 12 mg).

WHY PRESCRIBED
It is used to relieve symptoms of hay fever (allergic rhinitis) and other allergies that affect the upper part of the respiratory tract. These include sneezing, runny nose, and watering and itchy eyes.

CHILDREN'S DOSAGE
This depends on the severity of the symptoms and the age of the child. This product should not be given to a child under the age of twelve years without the advice and supervision of a physician. The usual recommended dosage is one capsule in the morning and one again in the evening, with a maximum daily dosage of 24 milligrams, but the prescribing physician may advise an individualized dosage.

PRECAUTIONS AND WARNINGS
This product should not be given to a child with asthma, glaucoma, or other chronic disorders without the advice and supervision of a physician.

POSSIBLE SIDE EFFECTS
The most commonly reported side effects include drowsiness, and (especially in children) excitability. More severe side effects are infrequent. An overdosage of antihistamine in infants and children can cause hallucinations, convulsions, and even death.

tetracycline (generic)

BRAND NAMES
Acromycin-V®, Minocin®, Panmycin®, Retet®, Robitet®, SK-Tetracycline®, Sumycin®.

PRODUCT CATEGORY
Antibacterial/antiamebic/antirickettsial.

DOSAGE FORM
Oral suspension, tablets, and capsules. Ophthalmic preparations are also available.

WHY PRESCRIBED
It is used to treat infections caused by a wide range of microorganisms, including certain species of bacteria, protozoa, and rickettsiae (intermediate in size between bacteria and viruses).

CHILDREN'S DOSAGE
This depends on the child's body weight and other factors. The usual total daily dosage of oral forms of tetracycline is 25 to 50 milligrams per kilogram of body weight (1 kilogram = 2.2 pounds), given in two to four equally divided doses. Tetracycline should not be given to children under the age of eight years unless the physician determines that other antibiotics would be ineffective or inappropriate.

PRECAUTIONS AND WARNINGS
Tetracyclines may cause permanent discoloration of the teeth if given to children under the age of eight years.

Do not give the child antacids while he or she is being treated with tetracycline since this could interfere with the effectiveness of the antibiotic.

Tetracycline should be used with caution (if at all) in children with impaired kidney or liver function.

POSSIBLE SIDE EFFECTS
The most common side effects include nausea, vomiting, diarrhea, heartburn, flatulence (gas), and loss of appetite (anorexia). Tetracyclines are capable of causing potentially more serious side effects in some patients, including damage to the blood-forming tissues and a severe generalized allergic reaction (anaphylactic shock).

Some children taking tetracycline, may experience severe skin eruptions and rashes when exposed to strong sunlight. These exaggerated "sunburn reactions" usually disappear days or weeks after therapy with tetracycline has been discontinued.

Theo-24®

GENERIC NAME
Theophylline.

PRODUCT CATEGORY
Bronchodilator.

DOSAGE FORM
Timed-release capsules.

WHY PRESCRIBED
It is used to prevent and relieve the symptoms of asthma and bronchospasm associated with chronic bronchitis.

CHILDREN'S DOSAGE
This product is not recommended for children under the age of twelve years. For older children, the dosage depends on several factors, including the *lean* body weight, age, frequency of doses, and severity of symptoms. The prescribing physician will individualize the initial dosage and may adjust it upward or downward according to the needs and response of the child.

PRECAUTIONS AND WARNINGS
Theophylline products should not be given to children who have a known hypersensitivity (allergy) to the drug. It also should not be used at the same time as other medications that may contain theophylline or a related substance. Caution should be used in giving caffeine beverages, including colas, or large amounts of chocolate to a child using theophylline medications. Theophylline may irritate the digestive tract of some children. It should not be given to a child with heart disease, hypertension (high blood pressure), thyroid disease, or impaired liver function without the advice of a physician.

POSSIBLE SIDE EFFECTS
Most side effects are associated with the use of doses that are larger than prescribed and may include nausea, vomiting (sometimes with bloody vomit), abdominal pain and cramps, headache, irritability, restlessness, nervousness, dizziness, and convulsions.

Theo-Dur®

GENERIC NAME
Theophylline.

PRODUCT CATEGORY
Bronchodilator.

DOSAGE FORM
Timed-release tablets.

WHY PRESCRIBED
It is used to prevent and relieve the symptoms of asthma and bronchospasm associated with chronic bronchitis.

CHILDREN'S DOSAGE
This product is not recommended for children who weigh less than 25 kilograms (55 pounds) and should be used in children under twelve years of age only with the advice and supervision of a physician. Because of variations in age, body weight, and severity of symptoms, the prescribing physician will individualize the initial dosage and may later adjust the dosage upward or downward according to the needs and response of the child to theophylline therapy.

PRECAUTIONS AND WARNINGS
This product should not be given to a child who has a known hypersensitivity (allergy) to theophylline. It also should not be given to a child who is already taking a medication that contains theophylline or a related substance. Caution should be used in giving caffeine beverages, including colas, or large amounts of chocolate to a child receiving theophylline. Theophylline should not be given to a child with heart disease, thyroid disease, hypertension (high blood pressure), or impaired liver function without the advice of a physician. Theophylline may irritate the digestive tract in some children.

POSSIBLE SIDE EFFECTS
Most side effects are associated with the use of larger than prescribed amounts of theophylline and may include nausea, vomiting (sometimes with bloody vomit), abdominal pain or cramps, loss of appetite (anorexia), headache, irritability, restlessness, nervousness, insomnia, dizziness, and convulsions.

Theobid®

GENERIC NAME
Theophylline.

PRODUCT CATEGORY
Bronchodilator.

DOSAGE FORM
Timed-release capsules.

WHY PRESCRIBED
It is used to prevent or relieve the symptoms of asthma or bronchospasm associated with chronic bronchitis.

CHILDREN'S DOSAGE
The exact dosage will be individualized by the prescribing physician according to several factors that include the age and *lean* body weight of the child, the severity of symptoms, and the frequency of doses. The initial dosage may be adjusted upward or downward by the physician after the needs and response of the child to theophylline therapy have been established.

PRECAUTIONS AND WARNINGS
Young children receiving theophylline should be observed closely for possible adverse effects since the child may not complain about the effects. The product should not be given to a child who is known to be hypersensitive (allergic) to theophylline. It also should not be given to a child who may be taking another medication that contains theophylline or a related substance. Caution should be used in giving caffeine beverages, including colas, or large amounts of chocolate to a child receiving theophylline. The drug should not be given to a child who may have heart disease, thyroid disease, hypertension (high blood pressure), or impaired liver function without the advice and supervision of a physician. Theophylline may irritate the digestive tract of some children.

POSSIBLE SIDE EFFECTS
Most side effects are the result of using larger than prescribed doses of theophylline and may include nausea, vomiting (sometimes with bloody vomit), abdominal pain or cramps, loss of appetite (anorexia), headache, dizziness, nervousness, insomnia, irritability, restlessness, and convulsions.

Theovent®

GENERIC NAME
Theophylline.

PRODUCT CATEGORY
Bronchodilator.

DOSAGE FORM
Timed-release capsules.

WHY PRESCRIBED
It is used to prevent and relieve the symptoms of asthma and bronchospasm associated with chronic bronchitis.

CHILDREN'S DOSAGE
This product is not recommended for children under the age of six years. Exact dosages vary because of several factors, including differences in the ages and *lean* body weights of children, severity of symptoms, and frequency of doses. The prescribing physician will individualize the initial dosage and may adjust it upward or downward according to the needs and response of the child to theophylline therapy.

PRECAUTIONS AND WARNINGS
This product should not be given to a child with a known hypersensitivity (allergy) to theophylline. It also should not be given to a child who is already taking a medication that contains theophylline or a related substance. Caution should be used in giving caffeine beverages, including colas, or large amounts of chocolate to children who are taking theophylline drugs. The drug should not be given to a child with heart disease, thyroid disease, hypertension (high blood pressure), or impaired liver function without the advice of a physician. Theophylline may irritate the digestive tract in some children.

POSSIBLE SIDE EFFECTS
Most side effects are due to the use of larger amounts of theophylline than prescribed and may include abdominal pain or cramps, nausea, vomiting (sometimes with bloody vomit), loss of appetite (anorexia), irritability, restlessness, headache, nervousness, insomnia, dizziness, and convulsions.

Thorazine®

GENERIC NAME
Chlorpromazine/hydrochloride.

PRODUCT CATEGORY
Major tranquilizer (plus sedative and antiemetic effects).

DOSAGE FORM
Syrup, oral concentrate, suppositories, and sustained-release "Spansule" capsules.

WHY PRESCRIBED
It is mainly used in children to treat severe behavioral problems, especially those characterized by explosive hyperexcitability and severe combativeness. Thorazine is also useful in the short-term treatment of children who are hyperactive and display various conduct disorders.

CHILDREN'S DOSAGE
This depends on the age, body weight, severity of symptoms, and the child's response to Thorazine therapy. The physician will adjust the dosage to the minimum amount that will provide control of symptoms.

PRECAUTIONS AND WARNINGS
This product should not be given to a child under the age of six months, except as a potential life-saving measure. It also should not be given to children, including teenagers, who show signs or symptoms of Reye's syndrome (a disease associated with a viral infection, such as chickenpox or influenza, resulting in damage to the brain and liver).

The drug should be used with great caution (if at all) in children with asthma or other disorders of the respiratory system.

POSSIBLE SIDE EFFECTS
Among the possible side effects associated with the use of Thorazine are skin rash, drowsiness, dizziness, blurred vision, constipation, dry mouth, hypotension (low blood pressure), rapid heartbeat (tachycardia), fever, jaundice (yellowing of the skin), and impairment of the blood-forming tissues. Children with epilepsy may also experience an increase in the incidence of convulsive attacks.

Tigan®

GENERIC NAME
Trimethobenzamide hydrochloride.

PRODUCT CATEGORY
Antiemetic.

DOSAGE FORM
Capsules and suppositories.

WHY PRESCRIBED
It is used to control nausea and vomiting.

CHILDREN'S DOSAGE
This depends on the severity of the symptoms and the body weight of the child. For example, the usual dosage for a child weighing between 30 and 90 pounds is one or two 100 milligram capsules, given three or four times daily. Pediatric suppositories are especially indicated for children who weigh less than 30 pounds.

PRECAUTIONS AND WARNINGS
The use of Tigan should be discontinued at the first sign of a skin rash or other evidence of an allergic reaction. Should this occur, consult the prescribing physician immediately.

Antiemetics, including Tigan, should be used only to control prolonged vomiting of a known cause. They should not be used to treat children with short-term, uncomplicated vomiting.

POSSIBLE SIDE EFFECTS
Some children may experience drowsiness, dizziness, blurred vision, muscle cramps, headache, and hypotension (low blood pressure). Less common side effects include jaundice, skin rashes, and impairment of the blood-forming tissues. In general, however, the incidence of side effects in patients taking Tigan is relatively low.

Tinactin® (OTC)

GENERIC NAME
Tolnaftate.

PRODUCT CATEGORY
Antifungal.

DOSAGE FORM
Topical cream, solution, and powder, and powder and liquid aerosol sprays. In addition, a Tinactin Jock Itch form is available as a cream and a spray powder.

WHY PRESCRIBED
It is used as a topical (applied directly to the skin) treatment for various fungal infections. These include athlete's foot (tinea pedis), ringworm of the body (tinea corporis), and mild fungal infections of the scalp (tinea capitis).

CHILDREN'S DOSAGE
Tinactin products are available without a doctor's prescription. Administer to children exactly as the label recommends.

PRECAUTIONS AND WARNINGS
Stop giving the child Tinactin at the first sign of skin irritation or possible allergic reaction, and consult the physician.

Do not apply Tinactin near the child's eyes. Be sure that the child does not inhale the aerosol forms of the drug.

POSSIBLE SIDE EFFECTS
Used as directed, Tinactin is relatively free from side effects.

Tofranil®

GENERIC NAME
Impramine hydrochloride.

PRODUCT CATEGORY
Antienuretic/antidepressant.

DOSAGE FORM
Tablets.

WHY PRESCRIBED
It is used in children six years of age and over to help reduce the frequency of bed-wetting (enuresis) when it is not associated with an organic (physical) disorder. The drug is also used to treat depression.

CHILDREN'S DOSAGE
This depends on the age and weight of the child. The physician will determine the dosage that best fits the needs of the individual child.

PRECAUTIONS AND WARNINGS
Tofranil should be used with caution (if at all) in children with heart disease, thyroid disease, or convulsive disorders (such as epilepsy). Because of the potential adverse effects of imipramine on the heart, the doctor may order an electrocardiogram before the start of therapy and at periodic intervals while the drug is in use.

POSSIBLE SIDE EFFECTS
The most commonly reported side effects in children include nervousness, fatigue, upset stomach and other digestive tract disorders, and disturbed sleep. Other side effects may be rapid heartbeat (tachycardia), sensation of heartbeat (palpitations), blood pressure changes, fainting, anxiety, emotional instability, and convulsions. These side effects often disappear as therapy continues or when the dosage is reduced by the physician.

Tolectin®

GENERIC NAME
Tolmetin sodium.

PRODUCT CATEGORY
Anti-inflammatory (nonsteroidal).

DOSAGE FORM
Tablets and capsules.

WHY PRESCRIBED
It is mainly used to relieve the symptoms of pain and inflammation associated with juvenile rheumatoid arthritis, rheumatoid arthritis, and osteoarthritis.

CHILDREN'S DOSAGE
This product is not recommended for use in children under the age of two years. For children age two and older, the total daily dosage depends on the severity of the symptoms and the child's age and body weight. The initial daily dosage is usually 20 milligrams per kilogram of body weight (1 kilogram = 2.2 pounds), given in divided doses three or four times a day. The physician may adjust the dosage upward or downward according to the needs and response of the child to Tolectin therapy.

PRECAUTIONS AND WARNINGS
Tolectin should not be given to children who are allergic to aspirin, especially if the aspirin induces symptoms of asthma or urticaria (hives).

Tolectin should be used with extreme caution (if at all) in children with disorders of the digestive tract.

POSSIBLE SIDE EFFECTS
The most commonly reported side effects include indigestion, abdominal pain and discomfort, nausea, vomiting, constipation, bleeding from the stomach or intestines, headache, skin rashes, drowsiness, and nervousness.

Triaminic® (OTC)

GENERIC NAME
This product contains a combination of phenylpropanolamine hydrochloride and chlorpheniramine maleate.

PRODUCT CATEGORY
Decongestant/antihistamine.

DOSAGE FORM
Tablets, chewable tablets, and syrup.

WHY PRESCRIBED
This product is used to relieve the symptoms of runny nose, nasal decongestion (stuffy nose), sneezing, itching of the eyes, nose, and throat, and watery eyes associated with the common cold, hay fever, and other nasal allergies.

CHILDREN'S DOSAGE
Although this product is available without a doctor's prescription, Triaminic tablets or syrup should not be given to a child under the age of six except with the advice and supervision of a physician. It should be used exactly as recommended by the label.

PRECAUTIONS AND WARNINGS
Do not give this product to a child who has hypertension (high blood pressure), thyroid disease, heart disease, asthma, glaucoma, or diabetes, or who is taking another medication without the advice and supervision of a physician. If symptoms do not improve within seven days, or if a high fever develops, consult a physician.

POSSIBLE SIDE EFFECTS
Triaminic may cause drowsiness or excitability in some children. Most side effects, particularly nervousness, sleeplessness, or dizziness, are the result of using larger than recommended doses of the drug.

Totacillin®

GENERIC NAME
Ampicillin.

PRODUCT CATEGORY
Broad-spectrum antibiotic (semisynthetic penicillin).

DOSAGE FORM
Capsules and oral suspension.

WHY PRESCRIBED
Totacillin is used to treat a wide range of bacterial infections in children, including those that involve the middle ear (otitis media), stomach and intestines (gastrointestinal tract), urinary tract, respiratory tract, the membranes that cover the brain and spinal cord (meningitis), and the skin.

CHILDREN'S DOSAGE
This depends largely on the severity of the infection and the child's age and weight. The site of the infection can also affect the dosage. For example, the usual dosage for children with an infection of the respiratory tract is 250 milligrams every six hours. However, if the child weighs less than 20 kilograms (44 pounds), the total daily dosage is usually 50 milligrams per kilogram of body weight (1 kilogram = 2.2 pounds), given in equally divided doses at intervals of six or eight hours. If kept refrigerated, ampicillin suspension usually remains stable for two weeks.

PRECAUTIONS AND WARNINGS
Totacillin should never be given to a child with a known allergic reaction to it or to penicillin. Adverse reactions are more likely if the child has experienced other allergies such as hay fever or urticaria (hives) or has asthma.

POSSIBLE SIDE EFFECTS
The most common side effects are diarrhea and skin rashes. Some children may also experience nausea and vomiting. More serious side effects are relatively uncommon.

Trimox®

GENERIC NAME
Amoxicillin.

PRODUCT CATEGORY
Broad-spectrum antibiotic (semisynthetic penicillin).

DOSAGE FORM
Capsules and oral suspension.

WHY PRESCRIBED
Trimox is used to treat a wide range of bacterial infections in children, including those that involve the ear, nose, and throat, urinary tract, skin, and lower part of the respiratory tract (air passages leading to the lungs).

CHILDREN'S DOSAGE
This depends largely on the severity of the infection and the child's age and body weight. The usual total daily dosage is 20 milligrams per kilogram of body weight (1 kilogram = 2.2 pounds), given in divided doses every eight hours. Be sure to shake the bottle well before giving the oral suspension.

PRECAUTIONS AND WARNINGS
Trimox should never be given to a child with a known allergic reaction to it or to penicillin. Adverse reactions are more likely if the child has experienced other allergies such as hay fever or urticaria (hives) or has asthma.

Long-term use of any antibiotic may result in the development of a "superinfection"—the growth and multiplication in the body of fungi and other species of microorganisms that are not affected by this product. Dispose of any remaining capsules or oral suspension once the course of therapy has been successfully completed.

POSSIBLE SIDE EFFECTS
Some children taking Trimox may experience diarrhea, nausea, vomiting, or skin rashes. More serious side effects are relatively uncommon.

Trind-DM® (OTC)

GENERIC NAME
This product contains in each 5 ml teaspoonful a combination of phenylpropanolamine hydrochloride (12.5 mg), dextromethorphan hydrobromide (7.5 mg), chlorpheniramine maleate (2.0 mg), and alcohol (5 percent).

PRODUCT CATEGORY
Antitussive (cough suppressant)/antihistamine/decongestant.

DOSAGE FORM
Liquid (fruit flavor).

WHY PRESCRIBED
It is used to relieve the symptoms of coughing, nasal congestion (stuffy nose), runny nose, sneezing, and itching, watery eyes associated with the common cold, hay fever, and other nasal allergies.

CHILDREN'S DOSAGE
Although this product is available without a doctor's prescription, the physician may prescribe the exact dosage based on the age and body weight of the child. The dosage may range from ⅛ teaspoonful every four hours for an infant over the age of three months up to 1 teaspoonful three or four times a day, as needed, by a child over the age of six years.

PRECAUTIONS AND WARNINGS
If the symptoms do not improve within three to five days, or if a fever develops, or the child has a persistent cough, discontinue using this product and consult a physician. This drug should not be given to a child with heart disease, hypertension (high blood pressure), asthma, diabetes, glaucoma, or thyroid disease without the advice and supervision of a physician.

POSSIBLE SIDE EFFECTS
Most side effects, including nervousness, dizziness, or sleeplessness, are usually the result of taking larger than prescribed doses of the drug. Some children also may experience drowsiness or excitability.

Tuss-Ornade®

GENERIC NAME
This product contains a combination of caramiphen edisylate and phenylpropanolamine hydrochloride. The liquid form also contains alcohol (5 percent).

PRODUCT CATEGORY
Antitussive (cough suppressant)/decongestant.

DOSAGE FORM
"Spansules" (timed-release) capsules and liquid (fruit flavor).

WHY PRESCRIBED
It is used to relieve coughing and throat irritation associated with the common cold and to loosen phlegm and mucus in the lower air passages.

CHILDREN'S DOSAGE

Age of Child	Teaspoonfuls (5 ml) Every Four Hours
2–6 years	1
6–12 years	2
12 years and over	3

Do not give Vicks Cough Syrup to children under the age of two years without the advice of a physician.

PRECAUTIONS AND WARNINGS
Prolonged coughing, especially if it is accompanied by fever or headache, may be a sign of a serious medical problem. In such cases, stop giving the child this product and consult a physician.

POSSIBLE SIDE EFFECTS
Used as directed, Vicks Cough Syrup is relatively free from side effects.

Valisone®

GENERIC NAME
Betamethasone valerate.

PRODUCT CATEGORY
Anti-inflammatory (synthetic corticosteroid).

DOSAGE FORM
Cream, lotion, and ointment.

WHY PRESCRIBED
It is used to treat various inflammatory disorders of the skin that are responsive to corticosteroids.

CHILDREN'S DOSAGE
The physician will give specific directions for use. In general, the ointment form of Valisone is used to treat dry or scaly areas of inflamed skin. If the inflamed area is moist, the cream or lotion forms of the drug are usually best.

PRECAUTIONS AND WARNINGS
Do not apply Valisone to areas of a child's skin that are infected. Not only does the drug have no beneficial effect on bacterial or fungal infections, but it may cause the disease to spread to nearby healthy areas of skin.

If Valisone causes local irritation of the skin, or if the inflammation seems to worsen, discontinue the use of the drug and consult a physician.

POSSIBLE SIDE EFFECTS
The most commonly reported side effects include itching, dry skin, skin eruptions, and a burning sensation at the site of drug application.

More serious side effects may occur if Valisone is applied to extensive areas of the skin and left on for prolonged periods. However, this is unlikely if the child is under close medical supervision and the physician's instructions are strictly followed.

Valium®

GENERIC NAME
Diazepam.

PRODUCT CATEGORY
Skeletal muscle relaxant/antianxiety agent.

DOSAGE FORM
Tablets.

WHY PRESCRIBED
It is mainly used in children to help relieve the symptoms of painful muscle spasms.

CHILDREN'S DOSAGE
This depends on the severity of the symptoms and the child's response to diazepam therapy. The usual starting dosage is 1 to 2.5 milligrams, given three or four times daily. The physician may gradually increase this dosage, when required, if the child does not experience troublesome side effects.

PRECAUTIONS AND WARNINGS
Valium should not be given to children under the age of six months. This drug should never be given to children unless it has been specifically prescribed for them by a physician.

Parents who are taking Valium for its action as a minor tranquilizer should never give a child their own tablets (the amount of active ingredient in the adult dosage form can be several times higher than that recommended for children).

POSSIBLE SIDE EFFECTS
The most commonly reported side effects include drowsiness, fatigue, and impaired muscular coordination (ataxia). At the dosage recommended for children for the control of muscle spasms, more serious side effects are relatively rare.

Vanceril®

GENERIC NAME
Beclomethasone dipropionate.

PRODUCT CATEGORY
Anti-inflammatory (corticosteroid).

DOSAGE FORM
Aerosol inhaler.

WHY PRESCRIBED
It is used in the treatment of bronchial asthma in children whose symptoms fail to respond to the usual types of bronchodilators and other nonsteroid medications.

CHILDREN'S DOSAGE
Vanceril should not be used for children under the age of six years. For children between six and twelve, the usual recommended dosage is one or two inhalations given three or four times a day, according to the needs and response of the child, but the total daily dosage should not exceed ten inhalations. Children over the age of twelve years are given the adult dosage of one or two inhalations three or four times a day, with a maximum of twenty inhalations in a single day. Rinsing the mouth after using an inhaler is recommended.

PRECAUTIONS AND WARNINGS
This product should not be given to a child who is known to be hypersensitive (allergic) to the drug. It also should not be used in the treatment of acute episodes of asthma or in a child who requires other corticosteroid medications only occasionally. If asthma symptoms persist during use of this drug, contact a physician immediately. Caution should be used in the administration of steroid drugs because of their potential adverse effects on the production of natural adrenal hormones.

POSSIBLE SIDE EFFECTS
Steroid drugs may cause a slowing of growth and development in children, and tend to suppress normal adrenal hormone production. Other side effects include dry mouth, hoarseness, and skin rashes.

V-Cillin K®

GENERIC NAME
Penicillin VK.

PRODUCT CATEGORY
Broad-spectrum antibiotic.

DOSAGE FORM
Oral solution and tablets.

WHY PRESCRIBED
It is used to treat a wide variety of bacterial infections.

CHILDREN'S DOSAGE
This depends on the severity of the infection, the type of bacteria involved, and the age and body weight of the child. For example, the usual total daily dosage for infants and small children is 25,000 to 90,000 units (15 to 56 milligrams) per kilogram of body weight (1 kilogram = 2.2 pounds), given in three to six divided doses. Penicillin VK is not as easily affected by stomach acid as is penicillin G. Thus, it is not necessary to take it on an empty stomach.

PRECAUTIONS AND WARNINGS
Penicillin should never be given to a child with a known allergy to it. Such hypersensitivity to the drug is greater in children who have experienced other allergies such as hay fever or hives (urticaria) or who have asthma.

Long-term use of any antibiotic may result in the development of a "superinfection"—the growth and multiplication in the body of fungi and other microorganisms that are not affected by the drug. Dispose of any remaining tablets or oral solution once the course of therapy has been completed successfully.

POSSIBLE SIDE EFFECTS
The most commonly reported side effects are upset stomach, abdominal discomfort or pain, diarrhea, a black "hairy" tongue, and drug-induced fever. In children who are hypersensitive to the antibiotic, penicillin can cause a severe and potentially fatal allergic reaction (anaphylactic shock).

Veetids®

GENERIC NAME
Pencillin VK.

PRODUCT CATEGORY
Broad-spectrum antibiotic.

DOSAGE FORM
Oral solution and tablets.

WHY PRESCRIBED
It is used to treat a wide variety of bacterial infections.

CHILDREN'S DOSAGE
This depends on the severity of the infection, the type of bacteria involved, and the age and body weight of the child. For example, the usual total daily dosage for infants and small children is 25,000 to 90,000 units (15 to 56 milligrams) per kilogram of body weight (1 kilogram = 2.2 pounds), given in three to six divided doses. Penicillin VK is not as easily affected by stomach acid as penicillin G. Thus, it is not necessary to take it on an empty stomach.

PRECAUTIONS AND WARNINGS
Penicillin should never be given to a child with a known allergy to it. Such hypersensitivity to the drug is greater in children who have experienced other allergies such as hay fever or hives (urticaria) or who have asthma.

Long-term use of any antibiotic may result in the development of a "superinfection"—the growth and multiplication in the body of fungi and other microorganisms that are not affected by the drug. Dispose of any remaining tablets or oral solution once the course of therapy has been completed successfully.

POSSIBLE SIDE EFFECTS
The most commonly reported side effects are upset stomach, abdominal discomfort or pain, diarrhea, a black "hairy" tongue, and drug-induced fever. In children who are hypersensitive to the antibiotic, penicillin can cause a severe and potentially fatal allergic reaction (anaphylactic shock).

Ventolin®

GENERIC NAME
Albuterol sulfate.

PRODUCT CATEGORY
Bronchodilator.

DOSAGE FORM
Syrup and tablets. An aerosol inhaler form is also available.

WHY PRESCRIBED
It is used to prevent and relieve symptoms of bronchospasm associated with obstructive airway disease.

CHILDREN'S DOSAGE
The syrup form of the product is not recommended for use in children below the age of two years. The tablets and inhaler are not recommended for children under the age of twelve years. The exact dosage is individualized by the prescribing physician according to several factors, including the age and body weight of the child and the severity of the symptoms. The physician may also adjust the dosage upward or downward after observing the needs and response of the child to a starting dosage.

PRECAUTIONS AND WARNINGS
This drug should not be given to a child with a known hypersensitivity (allergy) to the ingredients. Because the effects of Ventolin may last six hours or longer, additional doses, larger doses, or more frequent doses than prescribed should not be given. If the symptoms fail to improve or if they worsen, consult the physician. The doctor also should be consulted if the child is taking any other medication that may interfere with the action of Ventolin. The drug may aggravate a preexisting case of diabetes.

POSSIBLE SIDE EFFECTS
The most commonly reported side effects are nervousness and tremors, headache, rapid heartbeat (tachycardia), sensation of heartbeat (palpitations), muscle cramps, nausea, weakness, dizziness, insomnia, and difficulty urinating.

Vermox® Chewable Tablets

GENERIC NAME
Mebendazole.

PRODUCT CATEGORY
Anthelmintic (antiparasitic).

DOSAGE FORM
Chewable tablets.

WHY PRESCRIBED
It is used in the treatment of infections with whipworms (*Trichuris trichiura*), pinworms (*Enterobius vermicularis*), common roundworms (*Ascaris lumbricoides*), common hookworms (*Ancylostoma duodenale*), and American hookworms (*Necator americanus*), and mixed infections.

CHILDREN'S DOSAGE
This depends largely on the type and severity of the worm infection. For example, the usual dosage for children in the treatment of roundworms, hookworms, and whipworms is one tablet in the morning and one tablet in the evening, given on three consecutive days. Pinworm infections can often be controlled with a single dose of Vermox. In all such worm infections, a second course of therapy may be necessary after an interval of three weeks if the child is not cured.

PRECAUTIONS AND WARNINGS
Vermox should not be used in children with a known hypersensitivity (allergy) to the drug. It should be used with great caution (if at all) in children under the age of two years.

POSSIBLE SIDE EFFECTS
The only serious side effects are temporary abdominal pains and diarrhea associated with a massive infection and expulsion of worms.

Vibramycin®

GENERIC NAME
Doxycycline.

PRODUCT CATEGORY
Broad-spectrum antibiotic (synthetic derivative of oxytetracycline).

DOSAGE FORM
Syrup, oral suspension, capsules and tablets (Vibra-Tabs®).

WHY PRESCRIBED
It is used to treat infections caused by a wide range of microorganisms, including certain bacteria and rickettsiae (intermediate in size between bacteria and viruses).

CHILDREN'S DOSAGE
This depends on the child's body weight. The usual total daily dosage for children who weigh 100 pounds or less is 2 milligrams per pound of body weight, divided into two equal doses on the first day of therapy. On following days, the child is usually given half this amount, as a single daily dose or in two equally divided doses. Vibramycin (or other forms of tetracycline) should not be given to children under the age of eight unless the physician determines that other antibiotics would be ineffective or inappropriate.

PRECAUTIONS AND WARNINGS
Vibramycin (as well as other forms of tetracycline) may cause permanent discoloration of the teeth if given to children under the age of eight years.

Do not give the child antacids during treatment with Vibramycin, since this could interfere with the effectiveness of the antibiotic.

POSSIBLE SIDE EFFECTS
The most common side effects include nausea, vomiting, diarrhea, heartburn, and loss of appetite (anorexia). Potentially more serious side effects may include damage to blood-forming tissues and, severe generalized allergic reactions (anaphylactic shock).

Some children (as well as adults) taking Vibramycin may experience severe skin eruptions and rashes when exposed to strong sunlight. These exaggerated "sunburn reactions" usually disappear days or weeks after therapy with the drug has been discontinued.

Vicks® Children's Cough Syrup (OTC)

GENERIC NAME
This product contains in each 5 ml teaspoonful a combination of dextromethorphan hydrobromide (3.5 mg), guaifenesin (25 mg), and alcohol (5 percent).

PRODUCT CATEGORY
Expectorant/antitussive (cough suppressant).

DOSAGE FORM
Syrup (cherry flavor).

WHY PRESCRIBED
It is used to relieve coughing and throat irritation associated with the common cold and to loosen phlegm and mucus in the lower air passages.

CHILDREN'S DOSAGE

Age of Child	Teaspoonfuls (5 ml) Every Four Hours
2–6 years	1
6–12 years	2
12 years and over	3

Do not give Vicks Cough Syrup to children under the age of two years without the advice of a physician.

PRECAUTIONS AND WARNINGS
Prolonged coughing, especially if it is accompanied by fever or headache, may be a sign of a serious medical problem. In such cases, stop giving the child this product and consult a physician.

POSSIBLE SIDE EFFECTS
Used as directed, Vicks Cough Syrup is relatively free from side effects.

Vioform®-Hydrocortisone

GENERIC NAME
This product contains a combination of clioquinol (idochlorhyroxyquin) and hydrocortisone.

PRODUCT CATEGORY
Topical antifungal/antibacterial/corticosteroid (anti-inflammatory).

DOSAGE FORM
Cream, lotion, and ointment.

WHY PRESCRIBED
It is used to treat inflamed skin conditions such as eczema, infectious dermatitis, pruritus (itching) of the anal and genital areas, candidiasis, certain types of acne, and fungal infections that include tinea pedis (athlete's foot), tinea capitis and tinea corporis (ringworm), and tinea cruris (jock itch).

CHILDREN'S DOSAGE
Apply a thin layer of Vioform-Hydrocortisone to the affected skin areas three or four times daily. The physician may suggest the use of a mild form of either the cream or the ointment in treating less severe infections or when treating relatively large areas of the body.

PRECAUTIONS AND WARNINGS
Prolonged use of this drug may result in the growth and development on the body of microorganisms that are not affected by Vioform-Hydrocortisone.

Do not use this product to treat children who have chickenpox or other viral infections, since the drug may cause the infection to spread to healthy skin areas.

Do not apply the drug to large areas of the child's skin or leave it on for prolonged periods as this may increase the danger of adverse effects if the drug is absorbed through the skin.

POSSIBLE SIDE EFFECTS
Some children may experience a local irritation of the skin. Should this occur, discontinue using the drug and consult the child's physician immediately since it may be the first sign of an allergic reaction. Other commonly reported side effects include an itching and burning sensation, rashes, and dry skin.

Vistaril®

GENERIC NAME
Hydroxyzine pamoate.

PRODUCT CATEGORY
Sedative/minor tranquilizer/antipruritic (suppresses itching)/antiemetic.

DOSAGE FORM
Liquid (oral suspension) and capsules.

WHY PRESCRIBED
It is mainly used to help calm children who are emotionally disturbed, under stress, anxious, agitated, or apprehensive. The drug is also used to control nausea and vomiting (antiemetic action) and to relieve itching (pruritus) associated with certain skin allergies.

CHILDREN'S DOSAGE
The usual dosage for the control of anxiety and tension in children under the age of six years is 50 milligrams daily, given in divided doses. For children over the age of six, the dosage is between 50 and 100 milligrams daily, given in divided doses. The physician will adjust the dosage depending on the severity of the condition being treated and the response of the child to Vistaril therapy.

PRECAUTIONS AND WARNINGS
This drug should not be given to a child who has shown a hypersensitivity (allergy) to it. Do not give the child any other medicine at the same time as Vistaril without medical approval. Caution is recommended in use of this drug for prolonged periods; the physician should re-examine the child periodically to determine whether continued use of the drug is needed.

POSSIBLE SIDE EFFECTS
The most common side effect is drowsiness. Some children may also experience dryness of the mouth.

VoSol® Otic Solution

GENERIC NAME
This product contains in each milliliter acetic acid (20 mg), propylene glycol diacetate (30 mg), benzethonium chloride (0.12 mg), and sodium acetate (0.5 mg).

PRODUCT CATEGORY
Antibacterial/antifungal.

DOSAGE FORM
Solution (for administration directly into the outer ear canal).

WHY PRESCRIBED
It is used to treat infections of the external ear canal caused by microorganisms that are susceptible to the drug.

CHILDREN'S DOSAGE
Several drops of VoSol are applied to the the affected surfaces of the external ear canal after earwax and other debris have been removed. A cotton wick saturated with the product is inserted in the affected ear canal and allowed to remain for 24 hours. A few drops of VoSol are added to the wick occasionally while the wick is in place. After 24 hours, the wick is removed and 5 more drops of the drug are applied to the ear canal three or four times each day until a physician advises that the infection has been controlled.

PRECAUTIONS AND WARNINGS
The drug should not be used in a child who is allergic to it. The product also should not be applied to an external ear canal if the eardrum has been ruptured. If signs of irritation or other adverse effects are noted, discontinue use of the drug. The product is not effective against skin infections that may be caused by a virus.

POSSIBLE SIDE EFFECTS
Except for possible irritation or a stinging or burning sensation, no serious side effects are expected.

Wyamycin® E, S

GENERIC NAME
Erythromycin ethylsuccinate (Wyamycin E), erythromycin stearate (Wyamycin 5).

PRODUCT CATEGORY
Antibiotic.

DOSAGE FORM
Oral suspension.

WHY PRESCRIBED
Wyamycin is used to treat mild to moderate bacterial infections, especially when the child is known to be allergic to penicillin or when the bacteria do not respond to penicillin.

CHILDREN'S DOSAGE
This depends largely on the severity of the infection and the child's age and body weight. The usual total daily dosage is 30 to 50 milligrams per kilogram of body weight (1 kilogram = 2.2 pounds), given in divided doses three or four times per day. In treating particularly severe infections, the physician may double this amount.

PRECAUTIONS AND WARNINGS
Children should take erythromycin at the times and in the exact amounts prescribed by their physicians. Taking more than the prescribed amount is not only wasteful but can cause stomach discomfort, nausea, vomiting, and diarrhea.

Long-term use of any antibiotic may result in development of a "superinfection"—the growth and multiplication in the body of fungi and other microorganisms that are not affected by the drug.

POSSIBLE SIDE EFFECTS
Erythromycin is a relatively safe antibiotic. The most common side effects include urticaria (hives) and skin rashes, nausea, vomiting, diarrhea, and abdominal cramps and pains.

Wymox®

GENERIC NAME
Amoxicillin.

PRODUCT CATEGORY
Broad-spectrum antibiotic (semisynthetic penicillin).

DOSAGE FORM
Capsules and oral suspension.

WHY PRESCRIBED
Wymox is used to treat a wide range of bacterial infections in children, including those that involve the ear, nose, and throat, urinary tract, and lower respiratory tract (air passages leading to the lungs).

CHILDREN'S DOSAGE
This depends largely on the severity of the infection and the child's age and body weight. The usual total daily dosage is 20 milligrams per kilogram of body weight (1 kilogram = 2.2 pounds), given in divided doses every eight hours. Be sure to shake the bottle well before giving the oral suspension.

PRECAUTIONS AND WARNINGS
Wymox should never be given to a child with a known allergic reaction to it or to penicillin. Adverse reactions are more likely if the child has experienced other allergies such as hay fever or hives (urticaria) or has asthma.

Long-term use of any antibiotic may result in development of a "superinfection"—the growth and multiplication in the body of fungi and other microorganisms that are not affected by the drug. Dispose of any remaining capsules or oral suspension once the course of therapy has been successfully completed.

POSSIBLE SIDE EFFECTS
Some children taking amoxicillin products may experience diarrhea, nausea, vomiting, or skin rashes. More serious side effects are relatively uncommon.

Vitamins

Vitamins are a group of very complex and fragile substances that are essential in minute amounts for the normal functioning, growth, and development of the body. It is probable that not all vitamins have been discovered yet. Those that have been identified are traditionally classified as *fat-soluble* (A, D, E, and K) and *water-soluble* (all the rest, including the B complex vitamins and vitamin C).

Fat-soluble vitamins can be stored in body tissues, after being dissolved in fat before absorption through the walls of the intestinal tract. Excessive intake of vitamins A and D can be harmful; but, this is unlikely from the diet alone. The only natural foods that contain potentially toxic levels of vitamin A are the livers of bears and seals—hardly a standard mealtime delight for most people. However, parents should be cautioned that children can be poisoned by taking *excessive* amounts of vitamins A and D in commercially available multivitamin supplements.

The water-soluble vitamins cannot be stored efficiently in the body. Excessive amounts received in food or dietary supplements are normally flushed out of the body in the urine.

The routine use of dietary supplements—both vitamins and minerals (such as calcium, phosphorus, iodine, iron, magnesium, and zinc)—should be necessary only for those adults and children with an obvious deficiency that has been diagnosed by a physician. Nevertheless, some nutrition experts have challenged this previously firm position.

The traditional viewpoint is that children normally obtain all the vitamins and minerals they need—in addition to proteins, fats, and carbohydrates—in meals that are "well balanced." There is a general lack of understanding about what constitutes such meals in an age of convenience foods and fortified products. Some people feel a growing concern that many children (as well as adults) are being deprived of certain vitamins that are necessary to maintain good health. This may be possible for a variety of reasons.

For example, fragile vitamins in natural foods can be weakened or destroyed by commercial processing and preparation. In addition, it has been suggested that other factors can rob foods of their vitamin content, including soil depletion where food is grown, harvesting techniques, and prolonged storage.

Once food reaches the home, its vitamin potential can be reduced by lengthy storage in freezers, intensive heat or overcooking, and general lack of knowledge about how to obtain the maximum nutritional benefit. For instance, most of the vitamins can be left behind in the water when vegetables are boiled. In such cases, it would be nutritionally advantageous to drink the broth and throw away the limp vegetables.

Vitamins do not *directly* improve the general health of the body. There is no established medical evidence that they ward off infectious diseases (not even the common cold), provide energy, or make people feel better—despite the enthusiastic claims of some manufacturers of supplementary vitamin tablets and capsules. Of course, there is no doubt that a *prolonged dietary lack of specific vitamins* can lead to serious problems, most of which, fortunately, are virtually unknown today in the industrialized nations of the world. In countries with a low standard of living, meals may be grossly unbalanced and result in the emergence of diseases that are directly related to the lack of one or more vitamins. For example, a severe lack of vitamin C can cause anemia, spontaneous bleeding, and scurvy; a lack of vitamin D can result in rickets or softening of the bones (osteomalacia).

A word about the "well-balanced" meal is important. Experts on diet and nutrition tell us that it is important for health to have a well-balanced diet. However, in many cases the average parent is bewildered and confused by the conflicting approaches to food adopted in magazine and newspaper articles written by these "experts." The simple fact is that there is really no single dietary system or individual menu that can be said to reflect a diet that is universally well balanced for all people in all possible circumstances. What makes a balanced meal for a baby or child would not be appropriate for his or her father working in an office or factory or training for competitive sports.

At the same time, the human body is remarkable in its ability to obtain essential nutrients from a wide variety of foods. For example, people living in the tropics have subsisted for thousands of years on mainly starchy fruits and vegetables while fellow humans in frozen Arctic lands have depended largely on fatty animal foods, supplemented only rarely with fresh fruits or vegetables. While milk and eggs are regarded as ideal sources of proteins, they are avoided by strict vegetarians, who seldom suffer from their own diet. Nearly every subculture throughout the world prohibits one or more sources of nutrition that may be regarded as favored foods by members of other subcultures. Yet it is difficult to prove that one way of food selection is nutritionally superior to the other.

A degree of common sense is the starting point in making sure that the body is being supplied with adequate amounts of "fuel"—that is, taken collectively, food that is rich in the essential proteins, fats, carbohydrates, vitamins, and minerals. Too much of a single item of food in the diet, whether it be steak, grilled cheese, hamburgers, or anything else, cannot be a good thing. The keynote is *variety*.

Good health demands much more than vitamin supplements. Try to discourage children from eating too much "junk food" and offer them meals that include a generous amount of *fresh* fruits and vegetables. Nutritionally balanced and properly prepared meals should provide all the nutrients a child normally needs to be healthy and well. Choose foods that present an interesting variety of textures and flavors. The chart on pages oo-oo should give a good overview of vitamin food sources and the problems that result from deficiencies.

Vitamin Supplements

Multivitamin supplements are generally available without a doctor's prescription (the exception is basically limited to those multivitamins that also contain fluoride). However, it is a good idea to check with your doctor before giving a child supplementary vitamins.

Pediatricians and other physicians usually recommend *liquid* vitamin supplements for infants under the age of two years, particularly vitamins A, C, and D (often also including iron).

When you give children vitamin supplements, be sure that you follow the instructions on the label. Do not give a child more chewable tablets (or other dosage forms) than are recommended by the manufacturer.

Selecting from among the commercially available vitamin supplements can be extremely confusing, especially without the aid of a physician or other qualified health professional (such as your neighborhood pharmacist). The labels on many products are nearly unreadable without the aid of a magnifying glass. In addition, many multivitamin supplements also contain one or more minerals (especially iron), which may add to the cost of the product and not really be necessary for an individual child.

There is no easy answer to this often perplexing problem except to enlist the help and advice of the child's physician or a trusted pharmacist.

Many brands of multivitamin supplements for children are made in the form of chewable tablets that depict animals, monsters, or cartoon characters. The manufacturers have obviously designed their products to be visually appealing to children. This is all well and good, up to a point. But children should never be encouraged—directly or indirectly—to associate taking multivitamin supplements (or any other pharmaceutical product) with "candy," especially if the tablets contain *iron* (which can be harmful in large doses). Try to explain that they should never take their vitamins without adult supervision. Be sure to keep the bottles well out of reach of small children.

CHILDREN'S RECOMMENDED DAILY ALLOWANCES (RDAs) OF VITAMINS[1, 2]

Fat-Soluble International Units (IU)

Age	Weight Pounds	Weight Kilograms	Vitamin A	Vitamin D	Vitamin E
to 6 months	13	6	1400	400	3
6 months-1 year	20	9	2000	400	4
1 to 3 years	29	13	2000	400	5
4 to 6 years	44	20	2500	400	6
7 to 10 years	62	28	3300	400	7

[1] (Adapted from the 1980 revision of the Food and Nutrition Board, National Academy of Sciences-National Research Council, Washington, D.C.)

[2] Fat-soluble vitamins (A, D, and E) are traditionally measured in international units (IU). Water-soluble vitamins are measured in milligrams (mg), except for folic acid and vitamin B_{12}, which are measured in micrograms (mcg or ug).

These recommended daily dietary allowances provide for individual variations among most normal children as they live in

Choosing Vitamin Supplements

Some commercially available multivitamin supplements should not be given to children under the age of four years. Read the label carefully for specific instructions. (If necessary, buy a magnifying glass!) Other multivitamin supplements may be given to children who are at least two years old.

The labels on almost all multivitamin supplements for children will show the percentage of the Recommended Daily Allowances (RDAs) for specific vitamins. For children between the ages of two and four years, most multivitamin supplements provide an absolute minimum of 100 percent of the RDAs for ten important vitamins. The percentage of the RDAs for children over the age of four years is somewhat lower, although this varies with the individual vitamin. Again, check the label.

The chart below provides the Recommended Daily Allowances (RDAs) of the vitamins for children.

Water-Soluble (milligrams or micrograms)

C	Folic Acid	Thiamine	VITAMIN Riboflavin	Niacin	B_2	B_6	B_{12}
35	30	0.3	0.4	6	0.4	0.3	0.5
35	45	0.5	0.6	8	0.6	0.6	1.5
45	100	0.7	0.8	9	0.8	0.9	2.0
45	200	0.9	1.0	11	1.0	1.3	2.5
45	300	1.2	1.4	16	1.4	1.6	3.0

the United States under usual environmental stresses. Diets should be based on a variety of common foods in order to provide other nutrients for which human requirements have been less well defined.

Vitamins Available in Foods

Vitamins Essential For Good Health

Vitamin	Good Sources	Deficiency Results
A (retinol)	dairy products, liver, green leafy vegetables, yellow vegetables	retarded growth, reduced resistance to infection, dry skin, night blindness, eye disease
B_1 (thiamine)	wholegrain cereals, beans, peas, kidney, oranges, nuts, brewers yeast, fish, liver, pork, poultry, lean meat	nervous disorders, impaired digestion, colitis, loss of muscular coordination, paralysis, beriberi
B_2 (riboflavin)	eggs, liver, kidney, lean meat, green vegetables, wheat germ, milk, dried yeast	weakness, impaired growth, inflammation of the tongue, fissured lips, skin disorders, anemia, cataract, sensitivity to light
Niacin	lean meat, fish, dried yeast, beans, peas, whole-grain cereals, eggs	gastrointestinal disturbances, mental disturbances, pellagra
B_{12} (cobalamin)	liver, saltwater fish, dairy products oysters, kidney, lean meat (also produced by bacteria normally present in the digestive tract)	pernicious anemia

This table lists the most important vitamins, a selection of the best natural food sources, the types of problems that can result from true deficiency of a specific vitamin.

VITAMINS ESSENTIAL FOR GOOD HEALTH

Vitamin	Good Sources	Deficiency Results
C (ascorbic acid)	fresh fruits and vegetables, citrus juices (especially required for infants, as in orange juice)	lowered resistance to infection, tender joints, bleeding gums, anemia, scurvy
D (calciferol)	butter, eggs, liver, fish (salmon, tuna, sardines, herring), oysters, yeast	rickets, osteomalacia
E (tocopherol)	green leafy vegetables, margarine, wheat germ, lettuce, vegetable oils, wholegrain cereals	weakening and rupture of the walls of the red blood cells
Folic acid (folacin)	liver, yeast, green leafy vegetables	anemia
B_6 (pyridoxine)	meat, wheat germ, cereal grains, blackstrap molasses	nausea, vomiting, neuritis, skin inflammation around the mouth and eyes
Pantothenic acid (B complex)	eggs, nuts, liver, green leafy vegetables, beef, pork, lamb, chicken, herring, liver, bran, brewers yeast	no specific disease or disorder is known to be related to a deficiency
Biotin	liver, kidney, eggs, fresh vegetables	no specific disease or disorder is known to be related to a deficiency
K	leafy vegetables, beef, pork, cauliflower tomatoes, peas, carrots	spontaneous bleeding

Minerals

In addition to proteins, carbohydrates, fats, and vitamins, the body requires more than a dozen minerals in the diet to maintain a healthy state. Some of these minerals are needed in amounts that are so small that many people are surprised that they can have any effect at all (these are the "trace" elements). For the most part there is no need to worry about whether a child is getting enough minerals since a well-balanced diet supplies more than enough.

Among the three most important minerals obtained in the food we eat are iron, calcium, and iodine. Iron is needed for the production of hemoglobin, the oxygen-carrying pigment of the red blood cell. Calcium keeps the bones and teeth healthy and strong and plays an important role in the coagulation (clotting) of blood. Iodine is required in very small amounts for normal thyroid gland functioning.

Other minerals that are essential in the diet in varying amounts include the following: sodium (mostly in the form of common table salt), which helps regulate the fluid balance of the body; potassium, which plays a similar role to that of sodium; chloride, which is necessary for the formation of the digestive juice, hydrochloric acid, in the stomach; phosphorus, which, together with calcium, is an important constituent of bones and teeth; magnesium, which is essential in small amounts to help regulate body temperature and to aid in the process of muscle contraction (it also plays a role in the manufacture of proteins from amino acid, the "building blocks" of protein), and trace elements, such as fluorine (which is essential in the formation of bones and teeth) and copper (which acts together with iron in the manufacture of hemoglobin).

Representative Multivitamin Supplements for Children

The average supermarket or large drugstore may display dozens of multivitamin supplements, including some that also contain iron or other minerals. In general, all such products that are recommended for children contain ten essential vitamins: A, D, E (the fat-soluble vitamins); C (ascorbic acid); folic acid; thiamine (B_1); riboflavin (B_2); niacin, B_6; and B_{12}.

If the product is intended for use by children between the ages of two and four years, the label will clearly indicate this fact. Other multivitamin supplements are intended for use by children over the age of four years (as well as adults). In both cases the label will indicate the amounts of each vitamin and the percentage of the Recommended Daily Allowances (RDAs) that this represents.

For the age group between two and four years, it is standard practice to provide 100 percent of the RDAs for vitamins A and D and about 150 percent of the RDAs for the other eight vitamins.

In children over the age of four years (as well as some adults), the *same product* will generally provide 50 percent of the RDAs for vitamins A and E, 100 percent of the RDAs for vitamins D and C, and slightly lower percentages for the other vitamins.

Some multivitamin supplements provide extra amount of vitamin C—typically, over 600 percent of the Recommended Daily Allowance. If so, this will be clearly stated on the label—for example, "With Extra C." If the product also contains iron or other minerals, this fact will usually be reflected in the full name of the product (as in the examples of Flintstones Plus Iron or One-A-Day Vitamins Plus Extra C).

Dietary supplements of individual vitamins are also available, although they are usually not recommended for children unless a specific need has been suggested by a physician.

Multivitamin supplements that also contain fluoride are not available without a doctor's prescription.

Multivitamin supplements that contain iron can be harmful to children if they are taken in excessive doses. Thus, it is essential never to exceed the dosage instructions on the label or (if appropriate) the advice given by the child's physician.

Vitamins are vitamins. There is no significant biochemical difference between those that are "manufactured" (synthesized) in the laboratory and those that are obtained "naturally" from foods. The only practical difference is the cost and potency of specific brand-name products.

The following lists represent typical examples of multivitamin supplements (some also containing iron or other minerals) that are available for children. *These lists are offered only as representative examples of the dozens of commercially available products. In no way are they meant to suggest superior products.* If the potency and number of vitamins in a particular product are the same, it is wise to select the less expensive product. Again, vitamins are vitamins. There is absolutely no difference between two products that contain identical vitamins of equal potency.

The products listed here contain ten essential vitamins plus, when indicated by an asterisk (*), 15 milligrams of elemental iron:

Bugs Bunny Multivitamin Supplement
Bugs Bunny Plus Iron Multivitamin Supplement*
Flintstones Multivitamin Supplement
Flintstones Plus Iron Multivitamin Supplement
Poly-Vi-Sol Vitamins with Iron

Each tablet of the multivitamins in the list above provides the following quantities of vitamins and percentages of the Recommended Daily Allowances (RDAs):

% OF RECOMMENDED DAILY ALLOWANCES (RDAs)

Vitamin	Quantity	Ages 2-4	Ages 4 and Over
A	2500 IU	100%	50%
D	400 IU	100	100
E	15 IU	150	50
C	60 mg	150	100
Folic acid	0.3 mg	150	75
Thiamine	1.05 mg	150	70
Riboflavin	1.20 mg	150	70
Niacin	13.50 mg	150	67
B_6	1.05 mg	150	52
B_{12}	4.5 mcg	150	75
iron	15 mg	150	83

The following multivitamin products include extra amounts of vitamin C (ascorbic acid):
Bugs Bunny with Extra C Multivitamin Supplement
Flintstones with Extra C Multivitamin Supplement
Each tablet provides the following quantities of vitamins and percentages of the Recommended Daily Allowances (RDAs):

% OF RECOMMENDED DAILY ALLOWANCES (RDAs)

Vitamin	Quantity	Ages 2-4	Ages 4 and Over
A	2500 IU	100%	50%
D	400 IU	100	100
E	15 IU	150	50
C	250 mg	625	417
Folic acid	0.3 mg	150	75
Thiamine	1.05 mg	150	70
Riboflavin	1.20 mg	150	70
Niacin	13.50 mg	150	67
B_6	1.05 mg	150	52
B_{12}	4.5 mcg	150	75

The following multivitamin and mineral supplement, which is *not recommended for children under the age of four years,* is presented as a typical example:
One-A-Day Vitamins Plus Minerals
Each tablet of this type of product contains the following quantities of vitamins and minerals, with the percentages of the Recommended Daily Allowances (RDAs):

Vitamins/Minerals	Quantity	% of U.S. RDA
A	5000 IU	100%
E	15 IU	50*
C	60 mg	100
Folic Acid	0.4 mg	100
Thiamine	1.5 mg	100
Riboflavin	1.7 mg	100
Niacin	20 mg	100
B_6	2 mg	100
B_{12}	6 mcg	100
D	400 IU	100
Pantothenic Acid	10 mg	100
Iron	18 mg	100
Calcium	100 mg	10
Phosphorus	100 mg	10
Iodine	150 mcg	100
Magnesium	100 mg	25
Copper	2 mg	100
Zinc	15 mg	100

*15 IU meets the RDA for vitamin E established by the National Academy of Sciences.

In some cases, parents will note that multivitamin supplement labels indicate the percentage of Recommended Daily Allowances of vitamins (and minerals, if present) based on the needs of children aged 2-6 and 6-12 years. The following tables present typical examples of each daily dose of Monster (monster-shaped chewable multiple vitamins); and Monster With Iron (monster-shape chewable vitamins with iron) supplements.

Each Monster Multiple Vitamin Supplement Tablet supplies:

1 Monster MVS Vitamin	Quantity	% of RDA set by the NRC Ages 2-6	Ages 6-12
A	3500 USP units	140%	106%
D	400 USP units	100	100
C	40 mg	100	100
B_1	1.1 mg	122	92
B_2	1.2 mg	109	100
B_6	1.2 mg	133	100
B_{12}	5 mcg	333	250
Niacin	15 mg	125	94
Folic acid	100 mcg	50	33
Pantothenic acid	5 mg	*	*

* Recommended Daily Allowance (RDA) has not been established.

Each Monster with Iron Multiple Vitamin Supplement Tablet supplies:

1 Monster MVS Vitamin	Quantity	% of RDA set by the NRC Ages 2-6	Ages 6-12
A	3500 USP units	140%	106%
D	400 USP units	100	100
C	40 mg	100	100
B_1	1.1 mg	122	92
B	1.2 mg	109	100
B_6	1.2 mg	133	100
B_{12}	5 mcg	333	250
Niacin	15 mg	125	94
Folic acid	100 mcg	50	33
Pantothenic acid	5 mg	*	*
Iron	10 mg	100	100

* Recommended Daily Allowance (RDA) has not been established.

Here is another example of how some manufacturers present information on multivitamin supplements for children aged 2-6 and 6-10 years.

Pals (animal-shaped chewable multiple vitamins); and Pals Plus Iron (animal-shaped chewable multiple vitamins with iron).

Each (daily dose) Pals Multiple Vitamin Supplement Tablet Contains:

1 PALS Vitamin	Quantity	% of RDA set by the NRC Ages 2-6*	Ages 6-10*
A	3500 USP units	140%	106%
D	400 USP units	100	100
C	60 mg	150	150
B_1	0.8 mg	100	73
B_2	1.3 mg	145	108
B_6	1 mg	111	83
B_{12}	2.5 mcg	62	50
Niacin	14 mg	127	93
Folic Acid	50 mcg	100	66
Pantothenic Acid	5 mg	**	**

* Figures based on values for 6- and 10-year-olds.
** RDA not established. Made with natural sweeteners, artificial colors and flavors.

Each (daily dose) Pals Plus Iron Multiple Vitamin Supplement Tablet contains:

1 PALS+ Vitamin Tablet	Quantity	% of RDA set by the NRC Ages 2-6*	Ages 6-10*
A	3500 USP units	140%	106%
D	400 USP units	100	100
C	60 mg	150	150
B_1	0.8 mg	100	73
B_2	1.3 mg	145	108
B_6	1 mg	111	83
B_{12}	2.5 mcg	62	50
Niacin	14 mg	127	93
Folic Acid	50 mcg	100	66
Pantothenic Acid	5 mg	**	**
Iron	12 mg	120	120

* Figures based on values for 6- and 10-year-olds respectively.
** RDA not established. Made with natural sweeteners, artificial colors and flavors. KEEP OUT OF THE REACH OF CHILDREN.

Important Note to Parents

It cannot be overemphasized that dozens of excellent multivitamin supplements are commercially available. The examples given here are not intended to imply that any specific product is recommended. These products were selected at random to demonstrate the means by which various manufacturers present information on the potency of their vitamins and the corresponding percentages of the Recommended Daily Allowances for each.

If you feel that your child needs a multivitamin supplement, it is wise to shop around for the best value. Always remember that when the potency is equal, vitamins are vitamins.

List of Drugs by Primary Therapeutic Category

ANALGESICS (pain relievers)
Anacin
Anacin-3
aspirin
Bayer Children's Chewable Aspirin
Children's CoTYLENOL Chewable Cold Tablets
Children's CoTYLENOL Liquid Cold Formula
Children's Panadol
codeine
Congespirin Aspirin Free Liquid Cough Medicine
Congespirin Chewable Cold Tablets
Datril
Demerol
Dorcol Children's Fever & Pain Reducer
Liquiprin
Motrin
Nuprin
Pyridium
St. Joseph Aspirin for Children
St. Joseph Aspirin-Free for Children
Sinarest
Talwin

ANTIBIOTICS/ ANTIBACTERIALS
Amcill
amoxicillin
Amoxil
ampicillin
Augmentin
Azo Gantrisin
Bactrim Pediatric Suspension
Ceclor
Chlormycetin
Cleocin Pediatric
Dynapen
E.E.S.
E-Mycin
ERYC
Eryped
Erythrocin Stearate
erythromycin
Furadantin
Gantanol
Gantrisin
Keflex
Macrodantin
Minocin
Panmycin
Pathocil
Pediamycin
Pediazole
penicillin G
penicillin VK
Pentids
Pen-Vee K
Polycillin
Polymox
Principen
Retet
Robicillin VK
Robitet
Septra
SK-Ampicillin
SK-Erythromycin
SK-Penicillin VK
SK-Tetracycline
Sumycin
Tegopen
Tetracycline
Totacillin
Trimox
V-Cillin K
Veetids
Vibramycin
Wyamycin
Wymox

ANTICONVULSANTS
Dilantin
pheobarbital
Solfoton
Tegretol

List of Drugs by Primary Therapeutic Category (Continued)

ANTIDIARRHEALS
Donnagel
Kaopectate
Lomotil
paregoric
Pepto-Bismol
Rheaban

ANTIEMETICS/ ANTINAUSEANTS (motion sickness)
Antivert
Bonine
Dramamine
Emetrol
Marezine
Tigan

ANTI-INFLAMMATORY DRUGS
Cordran
Deltasone
Epifoam
Indocin
Kenalog
Lidex
Medrol
Meticorten
Orasone
Sterapred
Synalar
Tolectin
Valisone
Vanceril

ANTIHISTAMINES/ DECONGESTANTS
Actife
Allerest
Bayer Children's Cold Tablets
Benadryl
Children's CoTYLENOL Liquid Cold Formula
Chlor-Trimeton
Comhist
Congespirin Cough Syrup
Contac Jr.
Coricidin Demilets
Coricidin Medilets
Dimetane
Dorcol Children's Liquid Cold Formula
Dristan
Drixoral
Naldecon-EX
Neosypephrine
Nostril
Nostrilla
Novafed
Novahistine Elixir
NTZ Long Acting
Orande Capsules
Otrivin
Periactin
Phenergan Syrup
Rhondec DM Syrup
Sinex
Sudafed
Teldrin
Triaminic

ANTIPARASITICS / ANTIFUNGALS
Antepar
Eurax
Kwell
Lotromin
Monistat 7 Vaginal Cream
Mycelex
Mycelex-G
Mycolog II
Nilstat
Povan
Scabene
Tinactin
Vermox
Vioform-Hydrocortisone

List of Drugs by Primary Therapeutic Category (Continued)

ANTISPASMODICS
Bentyl
Combid
Donnatal
Librax
Robinul

**ANTITUSSIVES
(Cough Suppressants)**
Actifed-C Expectorant
Ambenyl Cough Syrup
Benylin Cough Syrup
Benylin DM
Calcidrine Syrup
codeine
Cremacoat
Formula 44
Glycotuss
Naldecon-DX Pediatric Syrup
Naldecon-EX Pediatric Drops
Nucofed
Robitussin
Robitussin-CF
Romilar Children's Cough Syrup
St. Joseph Cough Syrup for Children
Trind DM
Tuss-Ornade
Vicks Cough Syrup

**BRONCHODILATORS/
ANTIASTHMATICS**
Bronitin
Bronitin Mist
Bronkaid Mist
Bronkaid Tablets
Bronkotabs
Constant-T
Elixophyllin
Intal
Marax
Primatene Mist
Primatene Tablets
Proventil
Quibron
Respid
Slo-Bid
Slo-Phyllin
Somophyllin
Sultaire
Tedral
Theobid
Theo-Dur
Theo-24
Theovent
Ventolin

**DIETARY SUPPLEMENTS
(in addition to vitamins listed separately)**
Ferosol
Fer-In-Sol
Fero-Gradumet
ferrous sulfate
Lytren
Pedialyte
Poly-Vi-Flor

EMETIC
ipecac syrup

ENURESIS (bed-wetting) THERAPY
Tofranil

LAXATIVES / STOOL SOFTENERS
Agoral
Colace
Maltsupex
Metamucil
mineral oil

LOCAL ANESTHETICS
Baby Anbesol
Children's Chloraseptic Lozenges

List of Drugs by Primary Therapeutic Category (Continued)

MUSCLE RELAXANTS
Paraflex
Valium

OPHTHALMIC (eye) PREPARATIONS
Chloroptic-P S.0.P.
Cortisporin Ophthalmic
Isopto-Carpine
Neosporin
Sodium Sulamyd

OTIC (ear) PREPARATIONS
Auralgan
Cerumenex
Corticosporin Otic
Otic Domeboro
Vosol Otic Solution

SEDATIVES
Atarax
Butisol Sodium
Dalmane
Noctec
phenobarbital
Solfoton
Thorazine
Vistaril

Index

A

acetaminophen 24, 32, 72, 74, 76, 78, 82, 83, 87, 98, 101, 134, 169, 209, 213
acetic acid 167, 261
acetyl sulfisoxazole 121
Acromycin-V—*See* tetracyline 235
Actifed 21
Actifed-C Expectorant 22
activated attapulgite 198
Agoral 23
albuterol sulfate 193, 255
Allerest 24
aluminum sulfate 95
Ambenyl Cough Syrup 25
Ambenyl-D 26
Amcill 27
amoxicillin **28**, 29, 39, 187, 247, 262, Amoxil 29
ampicillin 27, **30**, 186, 192, 215, 246
Anacin 31
Anacin-3 32-33
Antepar 34
antipyrine 40
Antivert 35
aspirin 31, **36-37,** 44, 46, 207
Atarax 38
atropine sulfate 96, 97, 135
Augmentin 39
Auralgan Otic Solution 40
Azo Gantrisin 41

B

Baby Anbesol 42
bacitracin zinc 80
Bactrim 43
Bayer Children's Chewable Aspirin 44-45
Bayer Children's Cold Tablets 46
beclomethasone dipropionate 252
Benadryl 47, 58
Bentyl 48
Benylin Cough Syrup 49
Benylin DM Cough Syrup 50
benzethonium chloride 261
benzocaine 40, 42, 63
benzoic acid 98, 99
betamethasone valerate 250
Betapen VK—*See* penicillin VK 179
Bicillin—*See* penicillin 178
bismuth subsalicylate 182
bitartrate 190
Bonine 51

bromodiphenhydramine hydrochloride 25
brompheniramine maleate 93, 94
Bronitin Tablets 52
Bronitin Mist 53
Bronkaid Mist and Mist Suspension 54
Bronkaid Tablets 55
Bronkotabs 56
Butisol Sodium 57

C

Caladryl 58
calamine 58
Calcidrine Syrup 59
calcium acetate 95
calcium chloride 137
calcium iodide 59
CaldeCORT 60
caramiphen edisylate 249
carbamazepine 233
carbinoxamine maleate 206
Ceclor 61
cefaclor 61
cephalexin 128
Cerumenex Drops 62
cetylalcohol 108
cetylpyridinium chloride 214
chloral hydrate 157
chloramphenicol 64, 65
Chloraseptic Lozenges 63
chlordiazepoxide hydrochloride 132
chlorobutanol 62, 65
Chloromycetin 64
chlorpheniramine maleate 24, 66, 71, 78, 79, 82, 83, 99, 101, 161, 166, 213, 234, 245, 248
Chloroptic S.O.P. Opthalmic 65
Chlor-Trimeton Allergy Syrup 66
chlorpromazine 240
chlorzoxazone 172
Cleocin Pediatric 67
clidinium bromide 132
clindamycin palmitate hydrochloride 67
clioquinol 259
clotrimazole 136, 149, 150
cloxacillin sodium 232
codeine 59, **68**
codeine phosphate 22, 25, 163
Colace 69
Combid 70
Comhist 71

Index—283

Congespirin Aspirin-Free Cold
 Tablets 72
Congespirin for Children Cough
 Syrup 73
Congespirin for Children Liquid
 Cough Medicine 74
Constant-T 75
Contac Jr. 76
Cordran 77
Coricidin Demilets for Children 78
Coricidin Medilets for Children 79
Cortisporin Ophthalmic 80
Cortisporin Otic 81
CoTYLENOL (Children's) Liquid
 Cold Formula 82
CoTYLENOL (Children's) Chewable
 Cold Tablets 83
Cremacoat 84
cromolyn sodium 124
crotamiton 113
cyclizine hydrochloride 141
Cylert 85
cyproheptadine hydrochloride 183

D
Dalmane 86
Datril Extra Strength 87
Deltasone 88
Demerol 89
Desitin Ointment 90
dexbrompheniramine maleate 102
Dexedrine 91
dextroamphetamine sulfate 91
dextromethorphan 50
dextromethorphan hydrobromide 26,
 73, 76, 84, 118, 152, 204, 205, 210,
 248, 258
diazepam 251
dicloxacillin sodium 103
dicloxacillin sodium monohydrate
 174
dicyclomine hydrochloride 48
Dilantin 92
dimenhydrinate 100
Dimetane 93
Dimetane Decongestant 93
Dimetapp 94
diphenhydramine hydrochloride 47,
 49
diphenoxylate hydrochloride 135
disodium edetate 42
docusate sodium 69
Domeboro 95

Donnagel 96
Donnatal 97
Dorcol Children's Fever & Pain
 Reducer 98
Dorcol Children's Liquid Cold
 Formula 99
Dosage 14
doxycycline 257
doxylamine succinate 118
Dramamine 100
Dristin Advanced Formula 101
Drixoral 102
Dynapen 103

E
E.E.S. 104
edetate disodium 98
Elixophyllin 105
Emetrol 106
E-Mycin 107
ephedrine hydrochloride 52, 191, 231
ephedrine sulfate 55, 56, 140
Epifoam 108
epinephrine 53, 54, 190
ERYC 109
EryPed 110
erythromycin 107, 109, **112**
erythromycin ethylsuccinate 104, 110,
 176, 177, 262
erythromycin stearate 111, 216
Ethril—*See* erythromycin 112
Eurax 113

F
Feosol 114
Fer-In-Sol 115
Fero-Gradumet 116
ferrous sulfate 114, 115, 116, **117**
Formula 44 Cough Mixture 118
fluocinolone acetonide 229
fluocinonide 133
flurandrenolide 77
flurazepam hydrochloride 86
Furadantin 119

G
Gantanol 120
Gantrisin Pediatric Liquid 121
glycerin 40, 42
glycopyrrolate 201
Glycotuss 122
gramicidin 154

guaifenesin 22, 26, 52, 55, 56, 84, 122, 152, 153, 195, 203, 204, 258

H
hydrochloride 240
hydrocortisone 80, 81, 259
hydrocortisone acetate 60, 108
hydroxypropycellulose 130
hydroxyzine hydrochloride 38, 140
hydroxyzine pamoate 260
hyoscyamine sulfate 96, 97

I
ibuprofen 148, 164
imipramine hydrochloride 218, 243
Indocin 123
indomethacin 123
Intal 124
ipecac syrup **125**
isopropamide iodide 70
Isopto Carpine 126

K
kaolin 96, 127
Kaopectate 127
Keflex 128
Kenalog 129
Keralyt Gel 130
Kwell 131

L
Ledercillin VK—*See* penicillin VK 179
levulose 106
Librax 132
Lidex 133
lindane 131, 211
Liquiprin 134
Lomotil 135
Lotrimin 136
Lytren 137

M
Macrodantin 138
magnesium sulfate 137
malt soup extract 139
Maltsupex 139
Marax 140
Marezine 141
mebendazole 256
meclizine hydrochloride 35, 51
Medrol 142
meperidine hydrochloride 89

methylphenidate hydrochloride 199
methylprednisolone 142
Meticorten 143
Metamucil 144
miconazole nitrate 147
mineral oil **145**
Minocin 146
minocycline hydrochloride 146
Mol-Iron—*See* ferrous sulfate 17
Monistat 7 Vaginal Cream 147
Motrin 148
Mycelex 149
Mycelex-G 150
Mycolog II 151

N
Naldecon-DX Pediatric Syrup 152
Naldecon-EX Pediatric Drops 153
naloxone hydrochloride 230
neomycin sulfate 80, 81, 154
Neosporin Ophthalmic Solution 154
Neo-Synephrine 12 Hour Children's Nose Drops 155
Nilstat 156
nitrofurantoin 119, 138
Noctec 157
Nostril 158
Nostrilla 159
Novafed 160
Novahistine Elixir 161
NTZ Long Acting 162
Nucofed 163
Nuprin 164
nystatin 151, 156

O
Omnipen—*See* ampicillin 30
opium 68
Orasone 165
Ornade Spansule Capsules 166
orthophosphoric acid 106
Otic Domeboro Solution 167
Otrivin 168
oxymetazoline hydrochloride 155, 159, 162

P
Panadol (Children's) 169-170
Panmycin 171
Paraflex 172
paregoric **173**
Pathocil 174
pectin 96, 127

Pedialyte 175
Pediamycin 176
Pediazole 177
pemoline 85
penicillin G **178**, 180, 181, 200, 217, 253, 254
penicillin VK **179**
pentazocine hydrochloride 230
Pentids 180
Pen-Vee K 181
Pepto-Bismol 182
Periactin 183
Pfizerpen G—*See* penicillin 178
phenazopyridine hydrochloride 41, 194
Phenergan Syrup 184
phenobarbital 56, 97, **185**, 191, 223, 231,
phenolphthalein 23
phenylpropanolamine 24
phenylpropanolamine hydrochloride 46, 74, 76, 78, 79, 82, 83, 84, 94, 152, 153, 166, 204, 213, 245, 248, 249
phenyltoloxamine citrate 71
phenytoin 92
phenylephrine hydrochloride 71, 72, 93, 101, 158, 161, 214
pilocarpine hydrochloride 126
piperazine 34
Polycillin 186
polyethylene glycol 42
Polymox 187
polymyxin B sulfate 80, 81, 154
Poly-Vi-Flor 188
potassium chloride 137
potassium citrate 137, 175
potassium clavulanate 39
Povan 189
prednisone 88, 143, 165, 225,
Primatene Mist and Mist Suspension 190
Primatene Tablets 191
Principen 192
prochlorperazine maleate 70
promethazine hydrochloride 184
propylene glycol 62, 130
propylene glycol diacetate 261
Proventil 193
pseudoephedrine hydrochloride 21, 22, 26, 99, 160, 163, 206, 226
pseudoephedrine sulfate 102
psyllium hydrophilic mucilloid 144

Pyridium 194
pyrilamine maleate 52, 191
pyrvinium pamoate 189

Q
Quibron 195

R
Respbid 196
Retet 197
Reye's Syndrome 15-16, 31, 36-37, 44-45, 46 207-208
Rheaban 198
Ritalin 199
Robicillin VK 200
Robinul 201
Robitet 202
Robitussin 203
Robitussin-CF 204
Romilar Children's Cough Syrup 205
Rondec-DM Syrup 206

S
St. Joseph Aspirin for Children 207-208
St. Joseph Aspirin-Free for Children 209
St. Joseph Cough Syrup for Children 210
salicylic acid 130
Scabene 211
scopolamine hydrobromide 96, 97
Septra 212
Sinarest Tablets 213
Sinex 214
SK-Ampicillin 215
SK-Erythromycin 216
SK-Penicillin G—*See* penicillin G 178
SK-Penicillin VK 217
SK-Pramine 218
SK-Tetracycline 219
Slo-Bid 220
Slo-Phyllin 221
sodium acetate 261
sodium biphosphate 137
sodium butabarbital 57
sodium chloride 175
sodium citrate 137, 175
Sodium Sulamyd 222
Solfoton 223
Somophyllin-T 224
Sterapred 225
Sudafed 226

sulfacetamide sodium 222
sulfamethoxazole 43, 120, 212
sulfisoxazole 41
sulfisoxazole acetyl 177
Sumycin 227
Sustaire 228
Synalar 229

T
Talwin Nx 230
Tedral 231
Tegopen 232
Tegretol 233
Teldrin 234
tetracycline 171, 197, 202, 219, 227, **235**
Theo-24 236
Theo-Dur 237
Theobid 238
theophylline 52, 55, 56, 75, 105, 140, 191, 195, 196, 220, 221, 224, 228, 231, 236, 237, 238, 239
Theovent 239
Thorazine 240
Tigan 241
Tinactin 242
Tofranil 243
Tolectin 244
tolmetin sodium 244
tolnaftate 242
triamcinolone acetonide 129, 151
Triaminic 245
triethanolamine polypeptide oleate 62
trimethobenzamide hydrochloride 241
trimethoprim 43, 212
triprolidine hydrochloride 21, 22
Totacillin 246
Trimox 247
Trind-DM 248
Tuss-Ornade 249

V
Valisone 250
Valium 251
Vanceril 252
V-Cillin K 253
Veetids 254
Ventolin 254
Vermox Chewable Tablets 256
Vibramycin 257
Vicks Children's Cough Syrup 258
Vioform-Hydrocortisone 259

Vistaril 260
Vitamins 17-18, 188, 267
VoSol Otic Solution 261

W
Wyamycin E, S 262
Wymox 263

X
xylometazoline hydrochloride 168

Z
zinc oxide 90

Index—287

About the Authors

Edward R. Brace, a Fellow of the American Medical Writers' Association, has been a professional medical writer and editor for many years. He was formerly Associate Medical Editor at the Lahey Clinic in Boston and Medical Editor at two international drug companies. He is the author of *The Hamlyn Home Medical Guide,* was the Medical Editor of *The Good Housekeeping Family Medical Guide,* and has written and contributed to a number of other medical and related books—on both the technical and popular levels.

Kenneth Andersen has been a professional writer and editor of medical and scientific information for over thirty years. He is the author of *The Newsweek Encyclopedia of Family Health and Fitness* among many books, advisory editor of *Nutrition Today,* and for six years was editor in chief of *Today's Health* published by the American Medical Association. He studied medicine at the Northwestern University School of Medicine.